SMART CYCLING

SMART
CYCLING

Successful Training and Racing for Riders of All Levels

ARNIE BAKER, M.D.

A FIRESIDE BOOK
Published by Simon & Schuster

FIRESIDE
Rockefeller Center
1230 Avenue of the Americas
New York, NY 10020

First Fireside Edition 1997

FIRESIDE and colophon are registered trademarks
of Simon & Schuster Inc.

Designed by Irving Perkins Associates

Manufactured in the United States of America

10   9   8   7   6

Library of Congress Cataloging-in-Publication Data

Baker, Arnie.
     Smart cycling : successful training & racing for riders of all levels / by Arnie Baker.—
1st Fireside ed.
         p.   cm.
     "A Fireside book."
     Includes bibliographical references and index.
     (alk. paper)
     1. Cycling.   2. Cycling—Training.   3. Bicycle racing.   I. Title.
GV1041.B25   1997
     796.6—DC21   96-18734
         ISBN 0-684-82243-1   CIP

Optimist's creed reprinted courtesy of Optimists International.

First the women and then the men of Cyclo-Vets helped develop me as a coach. They changed my thinking and showed me that ordinary folks could be extraordinary athletes.

Contents

Part Four
RACING

Part Five
CYCLING IN YOUR HEAD

Acknowledgments

I have been helped by many, not only in the specific preparation of this book, but also in my development as a coach and as a racer:

Anne O'Brien and John Giroux for coaching me on the fundamentals of typography and desktop publishing. Jane Crossen and Joyce Copeland, who titled this book. Barbara Baker, Brian Begley, Kathy Feeney, Genna Mayberry, and Nelson Cronyn, who offered advice on and edited the early self-published editions.

Dan Lane and Sheila Curry at Simon & Schuster, who helped bring this book to a wider audience.

Mike Schnorr for illustrations and logo ideas.

Gary Leung and Gary deVoss for help with the articles on motivation and confidence.

I have benefited from my association with Ralph Ray not only in the exchange of many ideas, but in his product, technical, and mechanical engineering support.

Nelson Cronyn, who rode tandem with me—allowing me to show off some amazing heart-rate graphs and times.

Genna and Ron Mayberry for teaching me that goals are limited only by your imagination and that when bicycle parts "don't come that way" you can "make them or make 'em better."

Lee, John, Alan, and Ralph, who took me on my first fast rides and first taught me about bicycle training and racing.

Gary deVoss, who first introduced me to Cyclo-Vets and continues to encourage me more than a dozen years later.

Cyclo-Vets—my career bicycling club, whose members have helped me develop as a coach.

Carl Weymann and Adams Avenue Bicycles, Don Clark and La Mesa Cyclery—club and personal sponsors for more than a decade. Virgil Shrauner, whose Ultimate lightweight bicycle parts continue to astound.

I wish to specifically acknowledge Polar Electro Inc. for product help in heart-rate monitoring equipment and computer interfacing of data.

Gero McGuffin, who has helped not only in editing and criticism, but who rides with me every day.

Introduction:
Why *Smart* Cycling?

Many of us have learned the basics of riding a bicycle as children. The skills of mounting, balancing, braking, and changing gears seem relatively easy to learn. Even after years of being away from a bicycle, most of us can easily pick up riding again. "You never forget how to ride a bicycle" is a popular expression because, well, you don't.

Most of us know how to drive a car. Some of us remember the difficulties we faced when we were 16 and first took driver's ed or sat at the wheel next to a parent. Most of us don't give much thought anymore to the skills involved.

But in the back of our minds we know there are race car drivers with considerably more skills. We've heard about race schools, where "normal, mortal drivers" learn advanced steering, skidding, and speed skills There's a lot more to know.

Frankly, although many of us know a great deal about riding a bicycle, there is a lot more to know about training and racing. It's not necessary to know these things to ride a bicycle. But it is necessary if you want to race or train successfully.

You may have no intention of racing. You may never have thought of yourself as an athlete. You may have missed out on high school sports entirely. You are not alone.

No one in my family was the least bit athletic. I was always passed over when teams were picked in elementary school, and watched from the sidelines. I never played any high school or college sports. They called me, unkindly, "Arnie the spaz."

Even if you never plan to race, it's still fun and enjoyable to know how to ride well.

By learning the essentials of training and racing, by being a *smart* cyclist, you may find that you have a lot more ability than you ever gave yourself credit for. You may be surprised. I was.

SMART CYCLING

Part One

GETTING STARTED

CHAPTER 1

Bicycle Frame Fit

The right-sized frame is of paramount importance in assuring proper positioning on your bike. Proper position improves cycling efficiency, power, and comfort. In short, it makes you a better rider.

Frame Size Defined

The size of a frame is determined from the length of the seat tube. This is the tube that connects the bottom bracket to the seat. The size of frame you need relates most closely with the length of your leg.

The precise way in which manufacturers size their frames varies, but there are two generally accepted ways in which manufacturers measure frame size: Most road bicycles, with standard geometries, are sized by the distance along the seat tube from the center of the bottom bracket to the center of the top tube. This is called "center-to-center." Some bicycles are sized from the center of the bottom bracket to the top of the top tube. This is called "center-to-top." All measurements are made in centimeters. Bicycles such as Cannondales, with a seat tube that extends beyond the top tube, are sized differently.

Top Tube Length

The top tube runs horizontally from the seat to the headset. Although frame size (length of the seat tube) is the most important factor in choosing the frame that is right for you, different manufacturers have different length top tubes for the same size frame.

Women generally have shorter upper bodies and need a bike with a shorter top tube than men. Some adjustment can be made to the effective length of the top tube by choosing a handlebar stem with a longer or shorter extension. However, if your legs are very long or short in relation to the rest of your body, you may need to either pay special attention to the relative top tube lengths among manufacturers or consider a custom-built bicycle.

Seat Tube Angle

This is the angle formed by the seat tube and an imaginary horizontal line. For all-round road racing, a seat tube angle of about 73.5° is suitable. Hill-climbing specialists may desire a slightly slacker angle (a smaller degree). Crit riders may prefer a slightly steeper angle, 74° or 74.5°. Time trialists, duathletes, and triathletes prefer steeper angles, which give the rider a much more forward position. Some time-trial bikes are built with 80° seat tube angles. Most all-round road race bicycles are spec'd about right for general road racing.

Beginning racers will probably choose an all-round bicycle first. As your needs and riding style evolve, more attention should be given to the specific geometry of your machine.

Choosing Your Frame Size

The frame size you choose is directly related to the length of your inseam. This inseam measurement is not the same as your pant leg inseam. Follow the steps below to get the correct fit.

- First, determine your inseam measurement. Stand with your back to a wall with a 1-inch-thick book held between your legs, snug against your crotch. Measure from the floor to the top edge of the book.
- If you used inches convert to metric by multiplying by 2.54. One authority advocates a frame size 0.65 of inseam. He measures frame size center-to-center. Add 1.5 centimeters (cm) to convert to center-to-top.
- Another authority likes to see about 10 cm of seat post showing when the rider is mounted to know if the frame is the correct size. This, of course, requires an assembled bicycle. If you are buying a bike in a shop, this is a good way to check whether or not the frame size is right. A similar bicycle with similar components may be substituted if you are ordering a frame that has not yet been assembled into a bicycle.
- In general, when you stand over a road bicycle there should be 1 inch clearance between your crotch and the top tube in stocking feet, and about 1 to 2 inches with shoes.

CHAPTER 2

Position on the Bicycle

Now that you have determined the correct frame size, you must adjust the rest of your bike (seat height, stem height, pedal position, etc.) to ensure a perfect fit. The following general principles will help you achieve the correct fit, but remember that the final decision regarding position must be made by the individual rider. Optimal position is a compromise among many bicycling needs and may change depending upon the event since position affects muscle power, aerobic efficiency, comfort, and chance of injury.

Equipment

Bicycle, stationary trainer (if available), bike tools, plumb line, level, tape measure, calipers, and an assistant.

Setup

Set the bicycle level on a trainer, with the seat horizontal. If you don't have one, be prepared to take a spin around the block between adjustments.

Warm-up

Pedal moderately for at least 10 minutes before adjusting. Pedal moderately for a few minutes between adjustments.

Where to Start

The order in which you perform adjustments is important since some measurements are dependent upon others. The order outlined below works best for most riders.

Foot/Pedal Fore-Aft

The cleat of your cycling shoe should be positioned so that the ball of the foot is over the pedal spindle. Sprinters may prefer to back their feet out of the pedals a little more and be more on their toes.

Seat Height

Seat height is a compromise between aerobic efficiency, aerodynamics, power, comfort, bike control, and injury prevention. Cleat thickness, pedal type, and seat tube angle all influence this measurement. Formulas based upon inseam measurements or other body dimensions can only give approximate results and can only provide starting points.

The general idea is that the higher the saddle the more power you can generate and the less the aerobic cost, but don't become so far extended that your hips rock or your spin is restricted when you pedal. Higher positions are associated with back of the heel, back of the knee, or buttock discomfort.

A knee angle 25° less than a fully extended 180° is a good compromise between performance and injury prevention.

Seat Position Fore-Aft

Some riders position the seat fore-aft by measuring the distance a plumb line from the nose of the saddle falls behind the bottom bracket. Road riders tend to have the seat an inch or more back. Sprinters and time trialists tend to have a more forward position.

Other riders determine their seat position by dropping a plumb line from the front of their knees when the cranks are horizontal, and looking for the plumb to fall through the pedal axle.

For most 73.5° bicycles, road riders usually have their seats all the way back, time trialists all the way forward, and crit riders in between.

After you have adjusted the fore-aft position, repeat the determination of your seat height, since adjustment of saddle fore-aft may affect the seat height.

Seat Angle

Most riders ride best when the seat is level. Sprinters, aero time trialists, and women may have the noses of their saddles down slightly. Climbers may have their noses up slightly.

Foot/Pedal Rotation Angle

The cleat should be positioned so that your toes point nearly straight ahead. Some riders prefer their feet pointed slightly in, some slightly out. You may wish to ride a little with your cleats slightly loose, and see where you are most comfortable before final tightening. This adjustment is not as critical with free-rotation cleat systems that allow a certain degree of swivel rather than locking the foot into a fixed position. Free-rotation systems are thought to help decrease the chance of knee injury, but some riders still like to be locked in tight.

In general, if the outside of your knee hurts, adjust your cleats to point your toes a little more outward. If the inside of your knee hurts, point your toes a little more inward.

Handlebar Stem Height

The stem may be from 1 to 3 inches below the height of the top of your saddle. The lower your stem, the more aerodynamic you'll be. If your stem is too low, you may lose power or experience discomfort, especially in your neck, lower back, and crotch.

Stem Extension

Most bikes are sized so that most men end up needing stems with extensions of 10–13 cm. Most women use stems that are several centimeters shorter. When you are in the drop position there should be scant clearance between your elbows and your knees, and your back should be flat.

A rule of thumb is that the top of the handlebars should obscure the front axle when looking down with your hands in the drops.

Handlebar Shape

The shape of the handlebar varies with the type of riding. For general road riding, a long top horizontal section is preferred for climbing comfort. The drop of handlebars is partially determined by the comfort level of your hands in the curve.

Handlebar Width

Handlebar width should be roughly the width of your shoulders.

Handlebar Angle

The handlebars should be angled so that they are perpendicular to your seat tube. This means that they are pointed down about 15°.

Brake Levers

Brake lever tips are most comfortable when positioned such that their tips are in line with the bottom of the handlebar drops.

Toe Clips and Straps

Remember those? If you use them make sure that there is a small clearance between the tip of your shoe and the clip. Make sure the toe straps are at the outside edge of your shoes.

CHAPTER 3

Equipment Safety Checklist

Proper fit, proper installation, reliability, and maintenance of equipment are essential for rider safety and performance. Equipment must be clean, adjusted, and lubricated. Lightweight or aerodynamic equipment should not be used if it compromises safety. All riders should familiarize themselves with basic maintenance. No matter who works on your bike, you must check it and be confident of its safety.

Helmet and Gloves

These are vital pieces of safety equipment. They are necessary to race in many countries. Always wear a helmet when on any bicycle. Gloves not only make riding more comfortable, they protect your hands in case of a fall.

Helmet straps should be in good condition, not frayed, and adjusted for snug helmet fit.

Shoes

Cleats should be securely fastened and not overly worn. Check that Velcro, laces, or other closures are strong and functioning well.

Frame

Aligned, no cracks.

Wheels

No loose spokes. Rim is true. Wheel is aligned in frame and fastened tightly.

Tires

Check for hidden glass in tread. Replace tire if casing or sidewall cuts are present.

Sew-ups: Properly glued on, rim glue visible at edge. (See Chapter 5: Gluing on a Sew-up Tire.)

Headset

Adjusted without play. No "clicks" should be felt when steering.

Bottom Bracket

Adjusted without play. Rotates smoothly.

Crankset

Crank bolts tightened.

Brakes

Brake levers secure to handlebar—should be able to withstand moderate side pressure. Levers should return freely when released. Brake pads should hit entire rim surface simultaneously and flush.

Cables

Not frayed or torn. Cables slacken with time and should be tightened or replaced as needed. Tighten cables so that brake pads are a suitable distance from rim to ensure quick stopping power.

Seatpost and Saddle

Saddle aligned with top tube, all bolts tight.

Drivetrain

All gears working. Test on uphill grades or with pressure to assure cog/chain compatibility and to be sure gears do not change on their own. Adjust derailleur cable tension or tighten down tube shifter fixing bolt if gears change on their own.

Derailleurs adjusted so as not to shift into spokes or chainstay. (See Chapter 7: Adjusting Your Rear Derailleur.)

No stiff links in chain.

Handlebars

Securely fastened. Full body weight on the hoods, or aerobars if used, should not result in any slippage.

Handlebar plugs present.

Stem

Fastened securely. Aligned with front wheel.

Pedals

Check that cleats engage and disengage as desired. Clipless pedals: Adjust pedal tension if needed. Clipless pedals lightly lubricated.

Water Bottle Cages

Securely fastened. No cracks in welds or bends.

CHAPTER 4

Cleaning Your Bike

A clean bike looks good, and makes you faster as well. A clean, well-lubricated bicycle has less rolling and wind resistance. When you clean your bike, not only do you remove the dirt, you lubricate, inspect for damage, and replace worn parts.

What You Will Need

- Bucket
- Warm water
- Soap

- Degreaser (available at bike and auto-parts stores)
- Sponge(s)
- Brush(es)
- Tar remover (optional; available at auto-parts stores)
- Rags
- Chain lubricant
- Bike stand (if available)

Here's What to Do

- Place bike in the bike stand, or prop it up safely and securely.
- Give a filthy bike a preliminary water spray. Avoid moving parts, hub, bottom bracket, computer.
- Spray degreaser on the chain, chain rings, and freewheel. Avoid hubs, bottom bracket.
- Place a little detergent in warm water in the bucket.
- Sponge once over the frame, bars, and brakes to loosen dirt and remove the majority of it. Pay special attention to the underside areas of the bike.
- Wet the brush. Use it to clean the chain by rubbing it over the upper part of the chain while you use your hand to pedal backwards. This takes repeated wettings and several minutes. Special chain-cleaning devices are convenient and can work almost as well.
- Remove the wheels.
- Wet-brush the tires, rims, hubs, and freewheel.
- Use a rag to clean between the cogs of the freewheel, running an edge of the rag in the cog spaces.
- Check the wheels for loose or bent spokes and tire damage.
- Set the wheels aside.
- Sponge the bike more thoroughly, washing and cleaning all parts except your computer.
- Clean tarred areas with a sparse amount of tar remover.
- Sponge again with clear water.
- Inspect derailleur cables, brake cables, brakes, other bike parts.
- Wipe down the bike with a clean cloth, in part drying the bike, in part cleaning hard-to-reach places around the headset, brakes, crank axle.
- Replace the wheels and check that they are true.
- Lube chain by spraying lube into centers of jockey pulleys while hand-pedaling backwards.

CHAPTER 5

Gluing on a Sew-up Tire

Tires come in two basic types: clinchers or sew-ups. Each requires its own type of rim. The clincher system has a separate inner tube and outer tire. The sew-up, or tubular, with its integral tube sewed within the tire, is held to the rim with glue. Tubular tires are more expensive, more difficult to mount, and more difficult to fix. Although the gap is narrowing, tubulars have a performance edge—they are lighter, can be pumped to higher pressures, and offer better cornering performance.

How to Securely Glue a Tubular Tire to a Tubular Rim

Securely mounting a tubular prevents the tire from rolling off the rim with lateral forces. Serious crashes may result from a rolled tire.

Bicycles are subject to inspection at USCF events. Improperly glued sew-ups may result in rider penalties.

You may want to watch an experienced mechanic before attempting to mount your first sew-up.

What You Will Need

- Wheel
- Tire
- Tubular glue
- Truing stand (optional)
- Solvent
- Disposable latex gloves, plastic bag, or brushes
- Knife

Prepare the Rim

New rims may have a light coating of oil that needs to be removed with a solvent.

Previously used rims may have excess glue on their edges. A knife may be used to remove excess glue. By mounting the wheel in a truing stand and spinning the wheel, excess glue may be easily removed by rubbing the knife against the rim edges.

Stretch the Tire

All tubulars must be stretched to fit on the rim. If the unglued tire is easily stretched onto an unglued rim, you are ready to proceed.

Slightly undersized tubulars are almost impossible to mount without some extra stretching. To do this, stretch the unglued tire on a rim, inflate to 120 pounds, and leave overnight.

What Type of Glue?

Glues designed for tubular tires are traditionally clear or red. Use one or the other, but do not mix types.

Use about one tube of traditionally packaged sew-up glue per tire.

3M makes a car adhesive called FastTack. It comes in bigger tubes than sew-up glue, and costs less. It dries more quickly than traditional tire glues and you can ride on it sooner. It is, however, a little more difficult to remove a tire that has been mounted with FastTack.

Glue the Rim

There are several methods of gluing the rim.

A favorite is to set the wheel in a truing stand. Apply a bead of glue to the center of the rim, using about half a tube.

With the finger of a disposable-latex-gloved hand, spread the glue over the entire contact surface of the rim. Some use a finger covered by a plastic bag. It is important that the glue be spread over the entire rim bed, from rim edge to rim edge.

Another method is to use a toothbrush or other small brush to spread the glue.

If the rim is new, at least one extra coat is needed. Wait at least an hour, if not overnight, between coats.

Glue the Tire

Inflate the tire to about 40 pounds. It will fill and turn out, allowing the rim-strip surface to face up and be exposed. This makes applying glue to the tire easier.

Apply a bead of glue to the rim strip, using about half a tube. Spread the bead with a disposable-latex-gloved finger, plastic-bag-covered finger, or small brush. Spread over the entire rim-strip surface.

Glue smeared onto the tire surface does no harm and cleaning it from the tire surface with solvent may harm the sidewalls. Wipe off excess glue from the tire surface, but otherwise leave it alone.

Wait

The tire glue should be almost completely dry. The rim glue should be slightly tacky. (Note: I had you glue the rim first because it takes longer to dry.) An interval of 5 to 60 minutes may pass depending upon temperature and humidity.

Install the Tire

Deflate the tire, leaving just enough air for the tire to have some shape.

With valve hole up, place the rim on a clean, hard surface at ground level. Grass, dirt, or carpet surfaces are unsuitable—bits of material will stick to the glue.

Make sure the valve hole is clear of glue. Use a small twig or other item to clear the hole of glue.

Place the tire valve straight in the valve hole and grab the tire about 8 inches on either side. Push downward, stretching the tire, and slide your hands downward.

The last few inches are the most difficult. Lift the wheel. Place the valve side of the wheel into your chest for balance. Using your hands outstretched in front of you, work an edge of the tire over the rim edge, and then follow with the rest of the tire.

Once the tire is all the way on, inflate to about 40 pounds, and center the tire on the rim. The base tape should be showing evenly on both sides of the rim. Some brands center better with more pressure in the tire.

With tire pressure at about 40 pounds and with one hand on each hub edge, press the tire into the rim by rolling it along the ground, pressing down with your body weight. This helps remove air bubbles from the glue bed and helps maximize contact area.

Inflate the tire to 120 pounds. Wait at least overnight before racing.

In emergencies, some racers use FastTack'd rear tires after 1 hour if there are no sharp turns in their race. This may not be safe. It is certainly not safe for front tires.

Clean the Braking Surface

Use a solvent to clean the braking surface of the rim. Avoid the tire and carbon fiber wheel surfaces.

Checking Previous Work

It's good to see glue at the tire's rim edge. If you must roll back the tire to see glue, the job is suspect.

Apply moderate pressure and attempt to roll the tire off. It should not move.

A crackling sound indicates that the bond is dried out and that the tire should be remounted. It is usually, but not always, possible to remove a tire without damaging it. If the rim strip tears away from the tire casing, it is usually best to discard the tire.

CHAPTER 6

Lighten Your Bicycle

What do Greg LeMond, Pete Penseyres, Jane Fonda, and Jenny Craig have in common? They are all, sometimes excessively, concerned with weight. The first two were known as bicycle lightness freaks, each having bicycles in the neighborhood of 17 pounds.

Is Weight Important?

Look at riders who were always good on the flats but are now also climbing faster than ever before. Chances are their body or bike weight is down, and that accounts for part of their climbing improvement.

Figure a rider weighs about 157 pounds, and a bike about 23, for a total weight of 180 pounds. Since climbing is almost all work against gravity, consider a climber who sheds 6 pounds from his body, and 3 pounds from the bike, for a total of 9 pounds. That's about 5% less weight. In an hour's climb that is a savings of about 3 minutes, which can be the difference between winning and coming in 10th at a big stage race or the difference between making the lead pack and getting dropped in a road race.

I agree that if you are 20 pounds overweight, buying a lightweight bike may not be the answer. Don't let other riders tease you, though. Lightweight bikes are part of the answer. My own modified Trek 5500 weighs just over 14 pounds!

I'd like to discuss how to take weight off a bicycle. When discussing weight, I will refer to standard sizes, e.g., 56-cm frames, 170-mm cranks, 700c wheels.

Safety

As I stated previously, lightweight equipment should not be used when safety is the penalty. Reliability may occasionally be sacrificed for important events.

However, many modern lightweight parts are as safe as the heavy equipment they replace.

Weight Savings Made Easy

Saving weight on a bicycle used to be an esoteric art as there were only a very few manufacturers of truly lightweight parts.

The last few years have seen a tremendous increase in the availability of lightweight components. This is related to several factors:

- Mastery of new materials, especially carbon fiber and titanium.
- Decrease in aerospace manufacturing and the search for new markets by workers in that field.
- Increased availability of CNC (computer numeric controlled) machine tools, which have decreased the cost and increased the availability of custom parts.
- Increased market for lightweight parts, driven by the explosion in the mountain bike market.

Indeed, the lightweight after-market is a competitive one. There are many manufacturers of most of the lightweight parts described below. I have listed the names of a few manufacturers. Although the names in the future may change, the principles will not.

Weight Savings Not Costly

Riders who put together super-light bikes note that it costs about $1 per gram—or about $450 a pound—to save weight over standard components. Overall, that may be true, but there are plenty of places to get almost all of the weight savings and pay less than the standard costs.

Here's How

As our standard, let's pretend we are working with a steel racing bike with Shimano Ultegra STI components, and 32-hole Mavic MA40 rims. That's a bike almost any racer might be proud of, at 23.5 pounds, and costs over $2,000.

Remember, one ounce is 28.35 grams, and a pound is 454 grams.

FRAME SELECTION

"Steel is real," say the frame builders. Well, there is nothing unreal about titanium, carbon fiber, or aluminum, and a frameset weighs about 2 pounds less made from these materials. Years ago I rode a Vitus, a frameset weighing about 4.5 pounds, and less expensive than almost any racing steel frameset. Steel framesets weigh about 6.5 pounds. Many expensive titanium and carbon framesets are under 4 pounds. Several carbon brands are relatively inexpensive and weigh about 4.25 pounds.

Several carbon-frame bikes with Shimano Ultegra components are available at about $1,350. Right away you've saved $650 and over 2 pounds from our standard racing bike! What can we do with that extra $650? Do we even need to spend it all?

BOTTOM BRACKETS

An Ultegra bottom bracket weighs 287 grams. Titanium ones are about 160 grams—for a 125-gram savings at an extra cost of $125.

CRANKSETS

High-quality cranksets usually weigh about 650 grams. CNC cranks such as those from Topline are 4 or 5 ounces lighter—and cost an extra $110.

HANDLEBARS

Lightweight handlebars from Scott or TTT save 50 grams, almost 2 ounces over standard ones. Same price, or up to $10 more.

HANDLEBAR STEMS

A standard aluminum stem weighs almost 300 grams. Titanium stems—from Ultimate, Titus, Ibis, and others—weigh under 200 grams but may cost several hundred dollars more. Look around. Some chrome-alloy stems weigh only 250 grams, and cost the same as standard ones.

HEADSETS

Ultegra headsets weigh 142 grams. There are plenty of headsets costing the same that weigh 50 grams less. King headsets are not only lighter, they are better quality, though a little more expensive.

PEDALS

Lightweight pedals from Speedplay or Sampson weigh less than one-half the 470 grams of Ultegra clipless. Save 250 grams for no change in price.

HUBSETS

Ultegra hubsets weigh about 22 ounces. Use alloy or titanium cogs on lightweight hubsets from Ultimate, VeloMax, Zipp, or Nuke Proof and save 12 ounces. Costs about $150 more.

RIMS

Yes, Mavic MA40s are durable at 395 grams. But rims such as Sun Metal's Mistral 19A's are available at about 315 grams, for 160 grams saved a pair, no change in price.

SKEWERS

Lightweight hub skewers save 4 ounces for about $20 each.

SPOKES

Double-butted spokes, alloy nipples, 15 gauge instead of 14 gauge. You'll save about 3.5 ounces or 100 grams a wheel for about $25 more. If you need 14-gauge spokes because you're heavy, consider 14/16/14 butted instead of the traditional 14/15/14.

SEATS

A standard seat weighs almost 400 grams. Titanium rails are now popular and will give you a seat weighing 200 grams or less—for about $40 more.

SEAT POSTS

Seat posts come in titanium—for an extra $100. A lightweight alloy post by American Classic saves over 100 grams, no change in price. Titanium saves just 10 more grams.

BRAKES AND SHIFTERS

STI dual-pivot brakes offer great stopping power but a pair weighs in at a whopping 14 ounces. Hill climbers beware! A pair of lightweight brakes by CLB or Brew weighs just 7 ounces. Save 7 ounces on the pair. STI levers weigh over 21 ounces. Trade down to Shimano non-STI 105s, cheaper, great quality—save another 12 ounces.

DERAILLEURS

The sacrifice of index shifting is not worth the weight savings.

CHAINS

Lightweight drilled chains by Regina save 80 grams over Ultegra chains for $5 extra. Titanium chains are produced for a couple of hundred dollars and a savings of 80 more grams.

WATER BOTTLE CAGES

Standard bottle cages weigh about 45 grams. Look around. For the same price 20 grams can be saved with lighter cages.

CABLES

Hard-to-find alloy cables from CLB are $20 for a 100-gram savings. They stretch a little more than standard cables and mildly degrade braking performance, but braking is still very good.

NUTS AND BOLTS

Nuts and bolts are available in alloy or titanium. Weight is about half that of steel at a cost of $5 to $10 a bolt. Water bottle bolts, stem bolts, crank arm bolts, chain ring bolts, seat post bolts, even derailleur bolts and brake bolts are out there. Ultimate and SRP make hundreds of different ones.

Of Questionable Value

In our final tally let's ignore titanium chains, titanium stems, and titanium seat posts, which, for me, are too expensive for the weight saved.

Table 6–1

Part	Ounces Saved	Cost
Bottom bracket	4.5	$125
Brake cable	3.5	20
Brakes, levers	19.6	−100
Chain	2.8	5
Chain ring bolts	0.5	15
Cranks	4.5	110
Frame	36.0	−650
Freewheel	8.0	100
Handlebars	1.8	10
Headset	2.0	25
Hubs, cogs	12.0	150
Pedals	8.8	0
Rims	5.6	−10
Seat	7.0	40
Seat bolt	0.3	10
Seat post	3.6	0
Skewers	4.0	20
Spokes/nipples	7.0	20
Stem	1.4	0
Water bottle screws	0.3	10
Water bottle cages	0.7	0
Total, approximate	135 ounces	−$100

It All Adds Up

Keep in mind that a bike store might charge up to $50 in labor to change most of these parts, unless you are purchasing a new bicycle from them. You may wish to make these mods yourself, as parts need replacement.

The changes I have outlined add up to over 135 ounces, or about 8 pounds. As far as cost is concerned, these modifications will cost you about $100 less than our standard $2,000+ steel-framed bike. Your bike is down to 15 pounds. So I've done twice my part, and have saved you money at the same time. Now, it's up to you to just lose some of that fat!

CHAPTER 7

Adjusting Your Rear Derailleur

Adjustment of the rear derailleur seems to be a mystery to some riders. Knowing how is easy and an important step to bicycle maintenance independence. Since different wheels have different cog alignments, this skill is vital if you are constantly swapping racing and training wheels.

Range-of-Motion Adjustment

The rear derailleur needs limits to its range of motion. Without limits, it could overshift into your spokes when the derailleur cable is tightened, or shift into your frame's chainstays when released.

Figure 7–1

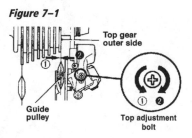

Top gear
outer side

Guide
pulley

Top adjustment
bolt

There are two little screws located on the back of most derailleurs. Looking from the rear of the bicycle, the top adjusting bolt usually governs the derailleur's motion for the smallest cog, and prevents the derailleur from traveling into the chainstays. Tightening it keeps the derailleur in toward the spokes, farther away from the chainstays. Loosening it allows the derailleur to travel out more, closer to the chainstays.

When tightening or loosening adjustment bolts, release any bolt tension that may be present on the derailleur. Do this by gently pressing the body of the derailleur toward the center cogs when you adjust this bolt.

With the rear derailleur cable loosened, look at the position of the jockey pulleys. Are they aligned directly under the smallest cog? If they are closer to the chainstays, tighten the bolt. If they are between the smallest cog and the next-smallest cog, loosen the bolt.

Figure 7–2

Pre-stretch
the cable
and remove
its slack

If your derailleur is new or being reinstalled, now is the time to fasten the dcrailleur cable. Cable adjusting barrels should be screwed in completely before you install cables. The derailleur adjusting barrel is located where the cable first reaches the derailleur.

Move the shifter forward to its position for the smallest cog. Connect the cable and tighten its fastening bolt. Use the shifter to increase cable tension, and shift back to the smallest cog. If the cable is now at all slack, loosen the bolt, reset the cable, and tighten the fixing bolt.

Figure 7–3

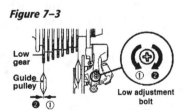

Now adjust the bolt governing low-gear adjustment. With the rear derailleur cable fully tightened, look from the rear and check the position of the jockey pulleys again. Too close to the spokes? Tighten the adjusting screw. Not over far enough and between the largest and next-largest cogs? Loosen the bolt.

Remember, bolts adjust most easily when not under tension. If you try to tighten this adjusting bolt with full cable tension, you are, in effect, trying to screw the bolt into the metal body of the derailleur.

Most people know that these two bolts adjust the range of motion of their derailleurs—but they forget which is which. No matter. Try one and watch what happens to the pulleys. Choose the wrong adjusting bolt? Fix it back to where it was and use the other one.

B-tension Adjustment

This is the little bolt that abuts a tab on the rear of the frame's dropout. This small derailleur bolt is technically called the B-tension adjustment bolt.

When the B-tension bolt is unscrewed, the derailleur sits closer to your freewheel. This results in more precise shifting. If you have a maximum of 21 teeth on your derailleur, this is where you want your derailleur. If you have up to 26 teeth on your largest cog, the derailleur needs to sit farther away from the cogset, or the jockey pulleys will rub on the larger cogs. Screw in the B-tension bolt to prevent this.

Index Shifting

Bicycles come with their rear derailleurs mounted. Most of the above adjustments have already been made. As cables stretch, however, or if you swap training wheels for race wheels, adjustment may be necessary. This is the adjustment that most riders need to know. It's easy.

The basic adjustment for index shifting is the cable adjusting barrel. This is located where the rear derailleur cable first passes into the rear derailleur.

With the front derailleur shifted to the big ring, and the rear shifter released, click-shift the derailleur one click. This should shift the rear derailleur to the second-smallest cog.

Look at the jockey pulleys. Has the shift been made? If not, the cable is not tight enough to shift, and you need to unscrew the SIS adjusting barrel by turning it counterclockwise.

If the jockey pulleys are well on their way to the third-smallest cog, you've overshifted and need to loosen cable tension by turning the adjusting barrel clockwise.

Try riding the bike. If your shifts to harder gears have a momentary delay before the shift is completed, you need to loosen the adjusting barrel, turning it clockwise. If the derailleur hesitates when shifting to an easier gear, or if it slips to a harder, smaller cog when climbing or sprinting, you need a little more cable tension. Tighten the cable by turning the adjusting barrel counter-clockwise.

Part Two

TRAINING

As an introduction to this section on training, the following is a list of 25 general hints to keep in mind during the course of your training regimen, whether you are a beginner or seasoned cyclist or are training indoors or out. Come back to this list for a quick reference every once in a while as a way of initiating a review of your overall program. The tips will help keep you on the right track.

- Get a plan, set goals, figure out what you need to get there.
- Keep a training log.
- Periodize your year, training differently during different seasons.
- Learn to work harder on hard days, easier on recovery days. Plan for recovery.
- Work on different aspects of fitness in different workouts.
- As a beginning cyclist, work on aerobics, endurance, and strength.
- As a seasoned cyclist, work on anaerobics, leg speed, and power.
- Work on strength with weight work, heavy gears, and one-legged riding.
- Join a club.
- Ride with riders both stronger and weaker than you are.
- Play intensity games with friends.
- Improve your riding technique and skills through practice and from coaches.
- Ride with relaxed, bent arms and with your knees in.
- Pull and push with the same-side hand and leg when climbing or sprinting.
- Establish a breathing rhythm when time trialing or climbing.
- Train in different riding positions.
- Use a heart-rate monitor.
- Wear a helmet and gloves, and keep your equipment safe and in good working order.
- Check your position on the bicycle, especially your seat height.
- Rely on food, not pills, for your nutrition.
- Maintain hydration by drinking before you are thirsty.
- Keep carbohydrate solution in your water bottle.
- Optimize your weight.
- Redirect the stresses in your life.
- Have patience with your program.

CHAPTER 8

Designing Your Training Schedule

Training Principles

The basic principles of a good training program are itemized below.

INDIVIDUALIZED

Athletes do not respond uniformly to training. Individualized training is needed to acknowledge this variability.

PROGRESSIVE

Your program should be progressive. Increased gains must be followed by increased demands. For example, as you are able to lift more weight, you must add weights to keep up with your growing strength.

DEMANDING

The program must be demanding. Your body must be overloaded in order to respond and adapt. Without overstimulation the body does not change and gains are not made. Without continual, persistent effort, the body will regress, atrophy, or even revert to a weaker state.

REPEATED

Repeating the same or similar workouts on a regular basis allows you to learn the demands of the workout and improve.

CHANGING

Repeating the same or similar workouts without variation leads to boredom and staleness. After you learn and master a workout or aspect of fitness, you should change or modify your program.

SYSTEMATIC

Your program must be systematic and well organized. A foundation is required. The development of certain body systems is required before other systems can be developed. For example, you can't squat heavy weights if your back doesn't have the development to support the weight. You can't perform repeated hard interval work without basic strength and some endurance. It's hard to train for sprints after a long hard day of climbing.

SPECIFIC

Specific training aimed at the specific development desired is paramount. The muscle groups and energy systems specific to the demands of your event must be simulated.

A bicyclist may have developed great leg strength and a great aerobic system, but as a first-time runner he will not be able to run close to his potential.

FLEXIBLE

The program must allow for deviation. It must, for example, allow for bad weather, illness, or other contingencies.

The program must allow the athlete, at least on some days, to work within ranges of intensity or duration that permit additional recovery or extra hard work.

MAINTAINED

Maintenance of fitness at a certain level requires less effort than was required to attain that level. After regression, restoration of the previous level of ability may take less time than if you were starting from scratch.

ASSESSED

Constant assessment of your program and appropriate goal setting result in faster and more consistent gains.

PERIODIZED

Your body is not a machine. Just as recovery is needed during a day's session of intervals, it is also needed in the long-range plan of the week, the month, the year, the cycle of years. Periods of more complete recovery during the winter, for example, allow the athlete to anticipate the coming year with renewed enthusiasm.

Strength and endurance work may compromise speed. By concentrating on strength and endurance during some periods and speed during other periods, overall development may be optimized.

Training must be seen within the broader scope of the athlete's long-range career and other priorities. The age-graded masters athlete may peak for racing at 50 or 51 years old, but may have backed off a little when 48 or 49.

FUN

Programs that lack fun or interest are usually not maintained. Even if it is physiologically appropriate, if it is too painful, boring, or complicated to perform, chances are you won't stay with it.

OVERTRAINING

If you place too many demands on yourself, overtraining may occur. Your body will not be able to respond and appropriately adapt. It will fail in one area or another, preventing further progress. Avoid overtraining.

Recovery, the readying of fitness systems to make further efforts, is discussed on page 36.

The Training Curve

The way from point A to point B is not a straight line! If you do not anticipate training curves, you may become frustrated and lose motivation.

TRAINING IS NOT LINEAR

Consider an athlete who is at a relatively low level of fitness, point A. The athlete would like to progress to a higher level, point B.

Training will not bring that athlete in a straight line from A to B. With the onset of training, the initial gains are great. But as training progresses, plateaus are almost always observed. Sometimes fitness even decreases.

Gains are made in spurts, in steps, rather than in a straight line.

By expecting and anticipating these steps, you will be less discouraged by apparent lack of progress.

Figure 8–1 **Training curve.**

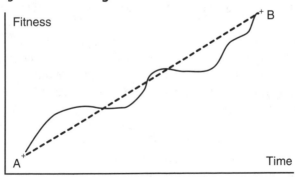

Typical training curves are steplike, as in the solid line—not straight, as in the dotted line.

This general rule applies during relatively short cycles of weeks and months, as well as with training over long cycles of years.

It applies to many other things as well—for example, it would also be typical for a weight-loss graph.

Bicycling Workout Variables

By understanding the variables of bicycling workouts you will understand how different workout programs function to achieve different ends and be better able to design your own.

The components of a bicycle workout can be broken down into five basic variables:

- Volume
- Intensity
- Cadence
- Position
- Pedal-stroke emphasis

These variables can be adjusted depending on the different goals you wish to achieve, whether it be improving your sprint or winning your first road race. Volume and intensity are standard workout variables that apply to almost any sport. Many riders and coaches neglect to consider that cadence, position, and pedal-stroke emphasis distinguish bicycling workouts and help train different aspects of fitness.

VOLUME

Volume is the total amount of work performed. In other words, it's the distance or amount of time you spend training in a given week, month, etc.

When work is performed in intervals, the length of each interval is called the duration of the interval. More information about interval training is found in Chapter 10.

Riding up to 200 miles or 15 hours a week helps improve aerobic and endurance fitness. Additional mileage primarily improves endurance.

Training for long road races requires time in the saddle to toughen the buttock tissues and adapt to riding position. Long rides, even those of minimal intensity, help train these needs.

INTENSITY

Intensity is the load or speed of work performed.

Perceived exertion, heart-rate monitoring, and the less commonly available power monitoring all have roles to play in assessing work intensity.

Heart-rate monitors help measure intensity, but they, too, are imperfect. If you work on leg speed, for example, and spin flat-out as fast as you can in an easy gear for 5 minutes, your heart rate may be very high, but your power output may be only moderate. More information about heart-rate training is found in Chapter 9.

On the other hand, if you sprint in a moderately hard gear for 20 seconds flat-out as hard as you can, your power output may be maximal, but your heart rate may not have time to "catch up" to a maximal effort.

Lactic acid levels in blood reflect anaerobic metabolism. They have been used as research tools in physiology labs for decades. Their use "in the field" is relatively new.

Power measurement—traditionally available on laboratory ergometers—is also available on new-generation portable "consumer" electronic stationary trainers. Force measuring devices can also be installed at the bottom bracket, pedals, or rear wheel axle.

As glycogen energy stores are exhausted, perceived exertion is relatively high compared with heart rate, lactic acid, or power levels.

CADENCE

Leg speed is another component of fitness.

Consider a rider told to work at a heart-rate intensity of 150 beats per minute for 15 minutes.

Those with a limited view of cycling fitness might think that if intensity and duration are defined, then the workout is determined. It is not.

Riding at 50 rpm in a big gear at a heart rate of 150 beats per minute (bpm) trains strength. Riding at 150 rpm at 150 bpm trains leg speed. The workouts are quite different and give different physical results.

Some fit riders can pedal very fast, but in an easy gear they are not necessarily working hard or going very fast.

POSITION

We all know that the leg muscles used in cycling are different from the leg muscles used in running. That's one reason why a good runner might be a lousy cyclist.

Within cycling, the muscles used in climbing are different from those used in flat riding. A position component is therefore part of the workout prescription.

Riding on the handlebar tops is often the best way to climb. That's because the legs have more power when the hip angle is open, and aerodynamics are of minimal importance when climbing.

Climbing in the drops slows you down as a climber. It's not what you want to do if you need to stay with the group on a climb. But it well may be what you want to do if you are training for more power in flat time trialing or crits!

Table 8-1 **Possible Workout Prescriptions Based on Type of Racing**

	Duration	Intensity	Cadence	Position
Sprinting	Short	Very high	Very high	Low
Criteriums	Moderate	High	High	Low
Road racing	Long	Moderate	Moderate	Mixed
Time trialing	Moderate	High	Low	Low
Climbing	Moderate	High	Low	High
Recovery	Short	Low	Low	Mixed

PEDAL-STROKE EMPHASIS

Athletes may appear to the casual observer to be performing similar work—this is not always the case.

Consider two athletes climbing for 5 minutes at 75% of maximum heart rate, at 50 rpm, on the tops of the handlebars. The athlete who concentrates on pulling up will be performing different work than the athlete who concentrates on pushing forward or who pedals smoothly.

Training with stroke emphasis—working specific muscle groups—defines yet another workout variable.

Periodization

Training is in part characterized by the five basic variables mentioned earlier. Periodization is how you shift these and other variables over the course of a week, month, year, or longer.

WHAT WE'RE TALKING ABOUT

We're talking about doing different things at different times. We're talking about varying workouts, about not doing the same workout every day. We're also talking about changing weekly schedules and changing monthly schedules during the year.

We're even talking about doing different things each year as an overall plan to improve ability.

COMMON TRAINING PERIODS

Our calendar divides the year into months, weeks, and days. On the simplest level, a periodized training program divides up a training year into similar periods of time.

The yearly cycle of racing (including local, state, and national championships), and yearly cycle of seasonal time change (wintertime loss of evening training hours, etc.), provides the basic large-training period.

A month is a convenient mid-length period of training.

Since most of us work Monday to Friday, and since many group rides meet on a weekly basis, the week is the basic small-training period for many of us.

LONGER TRAINING PERIODS

Other athletes see the sport in a larger frame of reference. Some elite athletes think of their long cycle as 4 years, coinciding with the Olympic Games. Masters athletes sometimes train in 5-year cycles, corresponding to age-graded 5-year age groups.

MACRO-, MESO-, AND MICROCYCLES

Instead of a frame of reference of year, month, and day, some coaches and athletes substitute *macro, meso* and *micro,* from the Greek meaning "large," "medium," and "small."

Athletes who periodize their training into 6-week blocks, for example, refer to a mesocycle of 6 weeks.

COACHING PHILOSOPHY

There are many ways to fit training into a weekly, monthly, or yearly cycle. You'll read and hear about different methods, different coaching philosophies, different things that work or don't. There are general principles. There is work that must be done in order to succeed. But there is no one right way.

PERIODIZATION UPS AND DOWNS

On the simplest level, we ride easy one day and go hard the next. We then recover before going hard again.

Figure 8–2

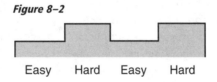

Easy　Hard　Easy　Hard

Such a graph might also apply to a monthly or yearly cycle. For example, some years we ride more and train harder; other years we get busy with family or work and reduce our riding.

As we try to fit rides into our week, a training graph might look a little more complicated:

Figure 8–3

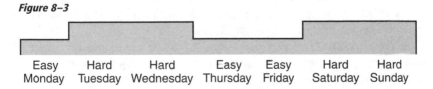

| Easy | Hard | Hard | Easy | Easy | Hard | Hard |
| Monday | Tuesday | Wednesday | Thursday | Friday | Saturday | Sunday |

Such a graph might represent a rider who has the time to ride hard two days in a row during the week and both days of the weekend.

BUILDING TO A PEAK

A more sophisticated training graph might have the following form:

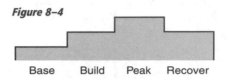

Figure 8–4

Base   Build   Peak   Recover

This common training graph can apply to training within a weekly, monthly, yearly, or longer training period.

It might represent the annual mileage of an Olympic athlete who builds annual training miles to a maximum the year before the Olympics and then tapers mileage to peak strength and speed during the Olympic year.

THE ANNUAL PLAN

Just as you need to allow time for adequate rest and recovery during your training week, your annual program needs modification from the specific daily training pursued during the racing season.

You can't train everything all at once. Significant increases in intensity, speed, and distance all at once are too demanding. When you work on one, you tend to lose a little in another.

You can incorporate what you need into an overall yearlong plan that will give you the right combination of strength, aerobic and anaerobic power, speed, and endurance during the racing season.

During the racing season, for example, you'd avoid beginning a serious weight program or markedly increasing your training distances. Both weight training and endurance are important parts in your success as a cyclist, but they rob you of the speed you need to compete successfully. You may need to incorporate these aspects of training into your plan at other times of the year.

RECOVERY

All of us need a period of relative rest during which we allow ourselves recovery from the racing season.

Rest may be needed, for example, to cure a case of chronic saddle sores. We may have home chores to accomplish, family and friends to pay attention to, money that must be earned and saved, and other obligations.

The racing season is a very busy time. After the racing season is over, but before we begin to prepare for the next racing season, is the time to allow for recovery and other chores.

Recovery does not mean partying and putting on 15 pounds. If you are under 10% body fat you can go up a few pounds. If you have weight to lose for next year, now is a good time to start getting rid of it.

The recovery period is a time of activity. You still ride and stay in some shape—though some forms of fitness are reduced. You may cross-train—skating, skiing, running, or performing aerobics. You may ride less than during the racing season, but ride at least a couple of days a week.

FOUNDATION

Once recovery has taken place, a foundation for the coming racing season can be laid. I believe the soundest foundation is one of strength and aerobic base. Aerobic base is more than just training the cardiovascular (heart and lungs) system. It's also training the muscles to take up and use oxygen. As the foundation period progresses, leg speed and endurance are added.

Weight training, bicycle touring, fixed-gear riding, and long group rides are part of this foundation period. Don't worry about how fast you are compared to your friends. Instead, use this time to develop a strong foundation and to work on individual and group riding skills in anticipation of the racing season.

PREPARATION

Preparation for the racing season includes the foundation elements described above and some anaerobic work.

This begins a period of intervals and sprints. Weight work and cross-training should be tapered to allow time for this more intense work.

RACING

The racing season demands a careful balance of the many elements of training.

Endurance and weight work continue to taper for most riders. Refer to the sections Weekly Training Schedule and Weekly Schedule by Days Available later in this chapter.

SPECIALIZATION

Sometimes riders want to peak toward a specific event.

For new racers this may be their big club race of the year. For others it may be their state or national championships. For a few in every country, it is the World Championships or Olympics.

Specialization involves a race-specific training program coupled with appropriate tapering for the big event.

For example, consider a rider who wishes to train especially for a criterium championship. Hill work is important for riders in all events because it builds strength and aerobic capacity. However, for this rider, hill work will be tapered to allow a greater emphasis on speed work. Race-specific interval work and motorpacing are workouts that may be added during specialization for this event.

Annual Periodization Chart

By varying distance, intensity, recovery, and specialized additional training such as weight work, a yearly cycle allows rest, development, and racing. Here's just one example of periodization.

Figure 8–5 **Annual periodization chart.**

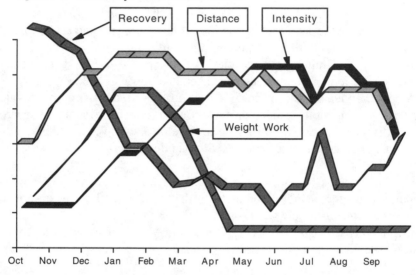

Note: This example is for a rider who lives in a southern U.S. temperate zone.

DISTANCE

Average miles ridden per week falls after the racing season. It rises during the winter months, building base and endurance, and falls slightly during the racing season. A taper in July for an important event results in a slight dip during that summer month, before picking up again in August, and then falling again in September and October as recovery begins again.

INTENSITY

Intensity is relatively low October through February. It then starts picking up and reaches a frenzy during the racing season, May through August. A slight taper in July allows extra recovery for peaking for a big event.

RECOVERY

The most time for recovery, and the most complete recovery, takes place in the period after the racing season—October and November. As miles increase and weight work becomes more intense, recovery is less.

A little extra recovery is allowed in July before the big event, but otherwise recovery awaits the end of the racing season once more.

WEIGHT WORK

Weight work begins gradually in October and reaches its peak in January and February. It falls away as the racing season picks up.

Weekly Training Schedule

Before the racing season arrives, it is important to plan carefully. You have only a limited amount of time, and must judge how to fit in the various kinds of training that you need.

WEEKLY NEEDS

Assuming that you are going to be a road racer this season, or want to train like one, let's consider what you need as far as training.

- Once a week, you need a race or race-type ride. This will be a hard ride, with flats, hills, and riding in a group with attacks.
- You need one day a week to practice sprints.
- You need an interval day.
- You need a longish endurance day at moderate pace.
- You need a day during the week of hills or at least partial hill work, in addition to your hill work on race/race-like day. Hills can be practiced in sprint, interval, endurance, or social rides.
- You need a rest day, possibly two. Not necessarily off the bike—perhaps a fun social day of riding without stress. This can be skill work at slow speed; for example, tumbling on the grass or practicing track stands.

GENERAL PRINCIPLES

- You can't go hard every day. You can build up to riding hard 2 days in a row.
- Interval days and race days should be your hardest days.
- Sprints are best done when you're relatively recovered and fresh.
- Resting 2 days before your hardest days, rather than the day immediately before, works best for most but not all riders. Riding moderately the day before helps prevent muscle stiffness.
- Train to race, not vice versa.
- Don't make the mistake of trying to "make up" for missed training sessions by combining too many activities into one day. This will only exhaust you for the weekend competition.

TRAIN SPECIFICALLY

- The best way to get strong in the sprint is to practice sprints.
- Intervals make you faster and stronger overall.
- The best way to be a good hill climber is to climb hills.

FITTING IT ALL IN

There are many different methods of establishing your weekly training schedule. There is no right way. Here's one way that seems to work for many.

Race day is usually Sunday. Two days before is Friday, so that should be a rest day. Monday is also a good day to rest after Sunday's hard ride or race.

The hardest non-race day is interval day. Interval day on Thursday works out well. That meshes with Friday as a rest day.

Sprint day is a short day, hard only for short periods of time. It does not take a whole lot out of you in terms of its effect the next day. Since many don't like to do sprints one day and intervals the next, many riders sprint on Tuesdays, leaving Wednesday as a moderate-paced endurance day or hill day.

For most of us who have regular jobs, Saturday is the club ride. That's a good place for a moderate social ride. Take it easy for the most part. Sure, you're with your friends and want to impress them. But you must keep track of your goals—it's silly to work so hard on Saturday that you can't keep up with Sunday's hard ride or race.

Table 8–2

Summary:		
	Sunday	Race
	Monday	Recovery
	Tuesday	Sprints
	Wednesday	Endurance, hills
	Thursday	Intervals
	Friday	Rest
	Saturday	Moderate

Weekly Schedule by Days Available

How might one organize the week with varying degrees of training time? There is no one right way. Here are some possibilities.

5 DAYS IF YOU CAN

If you wish to race and have a reasonable chance of being an all-round rider, 3 days of training a week is the minimum.

If you wish to race competitively, training at about the 5-day level will be necessary.

On Wednesday and/or Sunday, you could substitute about 1 hour of aerobics for 1 hour on the bike and have roughly equivalent workloads.

The training principles that have been used to give these suggestions could also be used to design many other valid programs.

Table 8–3

Day	Training Type	Mileage
3-Day Workout Schedule *(the minimum)*		
Tuesday	Sprints	20–25
Thursday	Intervals	30–40
Sunday	Race, race-like	40–65
Total		90–130
4-Day Workout Schedule		
Tuesday	Sprints	20–25
Thursday	Intervals	30–40
Saturday	Group ride	30–40
Sunday	Race, race-like	40–65
Total		120–170
5-Day Workout Schedule *(the ideal balance?)*		
Tuesday	Sprints	20–25
Wednesday	Endurance	50–60
Thursday	Intervals	30–40
Saturday	Group ride	30–40
Sunday	Race, race-like	40–65
Total		170–230
6-Day Workout Schedule		
Tuesday	Sprints	20–25
Wednesday	Endurance	50–60
Thursday	Intervals	30–40
Friday	Recovery or skill	15–25
Saturday	Group ride	30–40
Sunday	Race, race-like	40–65
Total		185–255
7-Day Workout Schedule *(so, you don't have a job?)*		
Monday	Recovery or skill	10–20
Tuesday	Sprints	20–25
Wednesday	Endurance	50–60
Thursday	Intervals	30–40
Friday	Recovery or skill	15–25
Saturday	Group ride	30–40
Sunday	Race, race-like	40–65
Total		195–275

Energy Systems

In order to work, muscles need energy. Understanding the body's different energy systems may help you understand training principles and help you make sure you have the fuel for work.

WHAT WE'RE TALKING ABOUT

The fuel for the body's energy production is food in the form of carbohydrates, fats, and protein. The food we eat is broken down by digestion and is used by the body to produce energy. How and when energy is produced has relevance to training.

ATP AND CREATINE PHOSPHATE

Adenosine triphosphate (ATP) is the fundamental source of the body's energy. All work, whether aerobic (with oxygen) or anaerobic (without oxygen), requires ATP.

ATP itself is stored in small quantities inside muscle cells. Another chemical, creatine phosphate (CP, also called phosphocreatine), also available within cells, provides a relatively quick, though limited, source of ATP.

The ATP and creatine phosphate found within cells can provide limited, immediate energy to working muscles. They do so without the presence of oxygen—that is, anaerobically.

Simple sugars, also found within cells, are used to make ATP. They can do so with oxygen (aerobically) or without oxygen (anaerobically).

When ATP is produced from simple sugars without oxygen, lactic acid is produced. Since lactic acid in high concentrations is toxic, the amount of simple sugars that can be used to produce ATP without oxygen is limited.

GLYCOGEN AND CARBOHYDRATES, FATS AND PROTEINS

The limited amount of stored ATP, creatine phosphate, and anaerobically produced ATP found within cells is sufficient for work that lasts up to 30 seconds.

Further energy must be obtained from the aerobic metabolism of the breakdown products of carbohydrates, fats, or proteins.

Ingested carbohydrates are broken down into simple sugars, principally glucose. Glucose may be formed into long carbohydrate chains within cells, a storage form of sugar called glycogen. When needed, the glycogen within cells can be broken back down to glucose.

Fats and proteins can also be converted to simpler substances to provide energy.

Although protein can also be converted to energy, the body tends to use proteins for other purposes—for example, muscle structure, enzymes, and transportation. Protein is used last as an energy source.

Up to about 2,000 calories of carbohydrates can be stored as glycogen.

Beyond that, excess carbohydrates and proteins are chemically converted to and stored as fat.

At relatively low intensities of work, most required energy is obtained from fats. As prolonged efforts become more intense, additional needs are met from glycogen.

As stated, the amount of energy stored in the body as glycogen is about 2,000 calories. Normally, this is sufficient for hard work lasting up to 2 or 3 hours. But very-high-intensity work can use up these calories sooner. About 50,000 calories are stored as fat in the average individual.

Once work reaches a moderately intense level, roughly the same number of calories from fat are used regardless of further training intensity. The additional calories required are supplied by glycogen.

Since bicycle racing is a high-intensity sport, an important element to success is the maintenance of glycogen stores through the ingestion of sufficient carbohydrates.

MONEY ANALOGY

The energy system is easier to understand if you use the money system as an analogy.

The basic unit of the energy system, ATP, is like money. The system demands its use for transactions. Immediate needs in the energy system are supplied by ATP and creatine phosphate. Immediate needs in the money system are supplied by coins and bills.

Relatively larger short-term needs in the energy system are supplied by anaerobic lactic acid production. In the money system, needs can be met by borrowing from credit cards. You've got a lactic acid and a credit card limit. And you've got to pay back your lactic acid or credit card debt.

Prolonged needs in the energy system can be met by energy production from aerobic reactions involving carbohydrates and fats. More prolonged needs in the money system come from savings—bank accounts, money-market funds, CDs, stocks, bonds, and property. Glycogen, the storage form of carbohydrate, is easily turned into energy. Fats are less accessible. Withdrawals from savings accounts and money-market funds are easy. Selling property can take some time.

There's a limit to how much energy can be reasonably produced—at which point more food must be eaten. There's a limit as to how much money you can spend before you have to find a job.

TRAINING ENERGY SOURCES

Energy systems can be trained. By training at a certain intensity, you can improve the energy systems needed at that intensity.

Understanding energy systems helps make the specificity and other principles of training understandable and logical.

CHAPTER 9

The Importance of Heart-Rate Monitoring

Why Use a Heart-Rate Monitor?

Heart-rate monitors allow you to observe your heart rate while working out. This has revolutionized modern approaches to training.

- Monitors are used in designing and implementing training and racing programs because they ensure that you work according to plan. A monitor helps make sure that you work hard enough. It also helps make sure that you don't work too hard!
- Monitors help analyze how you feel and what happens in training and in races. For some riders, monitors don't necessarily change training but allow an understanding of what is going on.
- Monitors help motivation. The feedback they provide is interesting and engaging for many riders.

MONITORS HELP ON GROUP RIDES

A big secret to training effectively is figuring out what you need out of a ride, then trying to get it. This is an area where a heart-rate monitor can be very useful.

Most club racers tend to follow along in club training rides or races, rather than being more demanding of themselves in figuring out what they need to do for their own training.

You can use a heart-rate monitor effectively when riding with other people if you allow it to let you know when you've slacked off too much and it is time to make more of an effort.

Say you're out on a steady endurance-paced ride. You are cruising in the pack, at a heart rate of 160. When the pace slows, so does your heart rate, say to 140. If your training goal is a high aerobic workout, you may not be using your time efficiently if you continue just to sit in. You must do something more to keep your heart training goal. And you can. You can go to the front and pull. You can spin an almost embarrassingly small gear, and your heart rate will rise (and your leg speed abilities too). You can attack the group.

MONITORS HELP ON SOLO RIDES

Most riders tend to train harder when with others, sustaining a higher HR. Many racers find that heart-rate monitors allow them to train alone more effectively.

You can use your heart-rate monitor to assure that you are putting into your interval workouts what you should. Most people should be able to achieve HRs over 90% of their maximum HR after hard 2- to 4-minute intervals.

Maximum Heart Rate

Determining maximum heart rate is the first step in developing a heart-rate training program.

WHY CARE ABOUT MAX HR?

For most riders, heart-rate zones for aerobic, threshold, and anaerobic work are based on their maximum HR. Many coaches and athletes attempt to determine max HR a few times a year in order to set training intensities.

Maximum heart rate is the highest heart rate you can achieve. For most riders, max HR is the highest accurate number they ever see on their monitor. I say *accurate* because sometimes electrical wires, radio transmitters, or other sources of false readings mess things up.

Session maximum heart rate is the highest heart rate during a particular exercise session. Few exercise sessions attempt to achieve a max, and so the session max HR is rarely near an individual's true max.

CONVENTIONAL WISDOM—NOT!

Conventional wisdom has it that your max HR, in beats per minute, is 220 minus your age. Conventional wisdom is a starting point, but not very accurate.

INDIVIDUALIZE YOUR NUMBERS

Taking 220 minus your age is useless. The statistical average for the population is useless for the individual. It's like saying the average person is 5'9" tall, so all bikes should measure 55 cm.

Cookbook figures are not only approximate but misleading. When I was 40 years old, by conventional wisdom, my max HR would have been (220 − 40 =) 180 beats per minute. Yet I routinely saw values between 195 and 200 in races and during maximal testing. I could time-trial above my so-called max for 40K. A 65-year-old woman I coach often sees 195 as her max.

MAX HR CHANGES

Max HR is not a static or fixed number. It is simplistic to say it is genetically determined.

People who are unfit may not be able to achieve their genetic potential because of a lack of muscular strength or energy to work hard. Their max HR will increase as they become fitter.

Once fitness exists, the maximum HR doesn't change much, but it does change. Elite athletes may actually have a lower max HR during their competitive seasons. And max HR is sport and climate specific. More on this follows.

DETERMINING YOUR MAX HEART RATE

To obtain a max HR value, you need to be:

1. Rested.
2. Well warmed up.
3. Motivated to make a maximum effort.

There are any number of different ways to find your max HR. Here is one way:

- Warm up for at least 5 to 10 minutes. After working at a moderate pace for 3 minutes, increase your effort by about 10% every minute. This means either increasing your cadence by 5 to 10 revolutions per minute or increasing your gearing by one gear of difficulty every couple of minutes.
- When you get to the point that it is extremely difficult to continue at pace, sprint absolutely as hard as you can for 30 seconds. Watch your heart monitor. This value should be close to your maximum.

Why rested? Rest provides for recovery from previous exertion. This may allow for repair of muscle microtears and resupply of glycogen. With muscle fatigue/soreness or a lack of glycogen, it is not possible to produce a maximal effort.

Why a warm-up? Max HR depends upon maximum cardiovascular demand. If you are not well warmed up, there's less blood flowing to your working muscles (the precapillary sphincters are not all open) so a maximum effort will not elicit a maximum response.

Why motivated? Many people only see their max in a race or a test in which they are really motivated. It's often difficult for riders to test their max when by themselves.

EFFECTS OF MUSCLE MASS, EXERCISE TYPE, AND POSITION

Some riders have had their maximum heart rate determined in other sports such as running or rowing.

Cardiovascular demand is proportional to muscle mass. Running uses more muscle mass than cycling or swimming and hence places higher cardiovascular demands on the athlete.

Body position may also affect cardiovascular demand. Horizontal position presents less demand than vertical position.

For these reasons your maximum heart rate is likely to be different for different sports. Your heart-rate training zones are likely to be different for swimming, running, and cycling. And they may even be different for time trialing or climbing.

Resting Heart Rate

Resting heart rate provides a tool for monitoring fitness and recovery.

MORNING RESTING HEART RATE

Resting heart rate is determined by counting or monitoring your heart rate while not engaging in physical activity. This is usually measured first thing in the morning while lying still in bed.

Conventional wisdom states that resting heart rate is a measure of fitness and recovery. As you get fitter, your resting heart rate falls. When you are not recovered, your resting heart rate rises.

Use resting heart rate as a tool in evaluation, but don't get spooked by high values: Some riders have their best performances on days when their resting heart rates are high.

FACTORS AFFECTING RESTING HR

Dehydration, fever or other illness, drugs, stress, or the environment might raise resting heart rate.

For many riders the discomfort of a full bladder, the physical activity of getting up to urinate, or the jarring of an alarm clock will raise heart rate. Resting quietly in bed for several minutes after returning from urinating or turning the alarm clock off will give a more accurate reading.

The value measured while lying flat on the back is often slightly lower than that measured while lying on the side.

OTHER RESTING HEART RATES

Although the morning resting heart rate is used by most, many believe that the resting heart rate recorded after lying quietly in bed for 5 minutes upon retiring in the evening is just as predictive of recovery.

The lowest heart rates occur during sleep. These values are obtained with a recording heart-rate monitor.

Still other athletes monitor standing resting heart rates. When you stand, your blood pressure falls. Sensors in the neck initially overcompensate for this decrease in blood pressure by sending signals that raise your heart rate. As the blood pressure returns to normal the heart rate slows, but remains at a level higher than the lying-down resting heart rate.

Some athletes monitor these changes in heart rate, believing them to be more sensitive indicators of recovery.

There are different techniques of evaluating these changes. One method is to observe the difference between lying-down resting heart rate and heart rate 1 minute after standing. This is called delta pulse. Another method is to observe the difference between heart rate upon standing and heart rate 30 seconds later.

Training may lower your resting heart rate. Even so, resting heart rate is, in part, genetically determined. Many racers whom I routinely beat are surprised that my resting heart rate is as high as 60.

Threshold Heart Rate

The heart rate that you can sustain for prolonged efforts is important in prescribing exercise training and as a measure of fitness.

TIME-TRIAL THRESHOLD

Here's a number that does matter: In a time trial (a steady-state solo race against the clock), what percentage of your maximum heart rate can you maintain?

Conventional wisdom has it that an athlete's time-trial threshold is about 85% of max HR. This may apply to beginning racers. Elite athletes have their time-trial threshold closer to 92% of max HR.

Percentages are more important than absolute number values. Ralph Myatt, a past national time-trial champ, used to time-trial at an HR of 140. During the same period of time I used to time-trial in the 180s. We both were riding at about the same percentage of our max, and we used to go about the same speed!

THRESHOLDS ARE VARIABLE

The concept of threshold training had its current popular bicycling origins with Professor F. Conconi's coaching of Francesco Moser for his hour record. For fit athletes, a threshold of 92% of maximum heart rate is relevant to events lasting about 1 hour. In bicycling, this corresponds most closely to a 40-kilometer time trial. For events longer than this, the threshold one can sustain will be lower. For shorter events, the threshold will be higher.

These percentages apply to well-rested, fit athletes, at moderate temperatures, at sea level.

LACTIC ACID AND ANAEROBIC THRESHOLDS

Physiologists mean something different by the term *threshold* than most bicycle riders do. Not only do many cyclists misuse these terms, but so do many coaches and cycling writers.

Lactic acid and anaerobic thresholds are defined in the physiology laboratory based on laboratory measurements.

Most cyclists have the notion that this is the same as time-trial pace. It is not. Time-trial pace, or time-trial threshold, is higher than the lactic acid and anaerobic thresholds that scientists determine in the laboratory.

Factors Affecting Heart Rate

A variety of individual and environmental factors affect heart rate. Interpreting heart rate in the context of these factors provides better insight into the meaning of heart rates.

TEMPERATURE AND HUMIDITY

Heat and humidity present increased demands on the body. To help cool the body, blood is shunted to the skin. This results in elevated heart rates.

Heart rates may be 1 beat higher for every 2 or 3 degrees above 70°F. Although submaximal and maximal heart rates are higher, power output with the exception of very short maximal sprint power—is reduced.

While some riders may need to expect higher thresholds when training, time trialing, or racing during conditions of heat and humidity, others will be so enervated that they are not able to perform or achieve their normal heart rates.

As in hot and humid conditions, cold weather also reduces power output. Cold weather results in lower heart rates.

ALTITUDE

Threshold and max HR are reduced about 1 beat for every 1,000 feet of elevation for athletes who have trained at sea level. For a given submaximal power output, heart rate is higher.

DEHYDRATION

Dehydration places increased demands upon the cardiovascular system. For any given power output, heart rates increase.

FITNESS

As non-elite athletes become fitter, they improve their cardiovascular function and increase their sport-specific muscle mass, thereby enabling themselves to achieve higher maximal heart rates.

As athletes become fitter they are able to produce more power for a given heart rate, or produce the same power with a lower heart rate.

As elite and professional athletes become fitter, they become more economical. In lay terms, their bodies are more efficient. Their muscle mass remains the same or slightly decreases. Their muscles work with less cardiovascular demand, and max HR may actually decrease during the racing season.

MEDICATIONS/DRUGS

Drugs may decrease or increase heart rate.

For example, beta-blockers—commonly prescribed for hypertension, migraine, and heart disease—lower the threshold and maximal heart rates.

Adrenergic stimulants found in decongestants or asthma medications raise heart rate. They can also cause heart irregularities—resulting in heart rates which can be misread by heart-rate monitors.

ILLNESS OR DISEASE

Medical conditions can decrease or increase heart rate.

For example, low thyroid function can decrease threshold and maximum HR. Conversely, hyperthyroidism can raise heart rate.

Heart-Rate Training Zones

You can establish heart-rate training zones based on percentages of your maximum heart rate. Different zone systems and many different coaching philosophies exist. A common heart-rate zone system is outlined here:

Table 9–1 **Heart-Rate Ranges/Zones**

	% Max HR	Effort
Noodling	<65%	Recovery, easy
Aerobic	66–85%	Club rides, warm-ups
Anaerobic threshold	86–92%	Time trials
Anaerobic		
Long	93–96%	Jumps, intervals
Short	97–100%	Sprints

NOODLING

Riding under 65% of your maximum heart rate. Easy riding. If your maximum is about 180 beats per minute, your noodling rate is under 120 beats per minute. This is recovery riding.

AEROBIC TRAINING

Working between 66% and 85% of your max HR. You are training aerobically. Aerobic means "with oxygen." This aerobic work will improve your ability to use oxygen efficiently.

Heart-rate economy will improve: As you become fitter, you will be able to accomplish the same work at lower heart rates. In other words, you will be able to accomplish more work at the same heart rate.

Recovery heart rate will improve: The fitter you are, the faster your heart rate will recover from hard efforts.

ANAEROBIC THRESHOLD TRAINING

Working between 86% and 92% of your max heart rate. You are at the border between aerobic and anaerobic work. This level of work is sustainable for efforts lasting up to an hour. This is the level at which you time-trial.

Threshold level will rise: New racers commonly sustain 86% of maximum heart rate. As fitness improves, levels closer to 92% of max heart rate can be maintained.

ANAEROBIC TRAINING AND RACING

In this range heart rate may be 93% or more of your max HR and can't be sustained for very long. This is very hard work. You get these efforts in jumps, intervals, and sprints. Red-line stuff. This is not the stuff most commuters, weekend riders, and century riders need to concern themselves with.

Training in this range is, however, vital for racers. Bicycling is an anaerobic sport—stuff like breakaways and the dropping of riders only happens when at least some racers are anaerobic or max'd out.

Efforts of this intensity preceded by periods of recovery may not result in heart rates over 93% of max HR. You must already be riding at high aerobic levels for these anaerobic efforts to result in very high heart rates. Remember that all efforts at heart rates above 93% of max are anaerobic, but not all anaerobic efforts will result in this high a heart rate.

THE EXERCISE PRESCRIPTION

All of the heart-rate zones on page 52 are sport and climate specific. Percentage intensity zones apply to the conditions under which the maximum was determined. When conditions change, maximum heart rate changes, and so the various zones must be reassessed.

TRAINING TIME NEEDED TO PROGRESS

To train the aerobic system, I believe riders need high-aerobic work—80% to 85% of maximum heart rate—for at least 30 minutes, three times a week. It would also probably be best to ride at 80–85% of max HR for at least an hour at least once a week.

Racers also need threshold work—85–92% of maximum HR—as well as anaerobic work—over 93% of maximum HR—during these periods. This may not necessarily be a "training ride," it may be race day. Of course, racing is training.

As racers move up in ability categories, their races become longer. They need more endurance and more ability to respond to repeated attacks. They still need high-aerobic work, but the percentage of time they spend in the

Table 9-2 **Training Heart-Rate Guidelines**

Max HR (beats per min.)	Aerobic (66–85%)	Threshold (86–92%)	Anaerobic (93+%)
205	135–174	175–189	190
200	132–170	171–184	185
195	129–166	167–179	180
190	125–162	163–175	176
185	122–157	158–170	171
180	119–153	154–166	167
175	116–149	150–161	162
170	112–145	146–156	157
165	109–140	141–152	153
160	106–136	137–147	148
155	102–132	133–143	144
150	99–128	129–138	139

high-aerobic range decreases. They spend more time at opposite ends of the percentage scale: in the low-aerobic range and in the anaerobic range.

Heart-Rate Training Isn't Everything

Although heart-rate monitoring has revolutionized training for many, it's not a be-all and end-all. While heart rate is one measure of training intensity, it's not always the appropriate way to measure intensity. Not everyone finds that heart-rate monitoring improves performance. And not everyone can figure out the buttons or process the data.

HEART TRAINING IS SPECIFIC

When you are training, you must consider the purpose of your training. Are you training to get the maximum heart workout? Are you training to get the maximum leg strength? Are you training to ride the fastest you can right now?

Training may involve targeting the heart or the legs—in different parts of the same session, in different sessions, or at the same time.

"INEFFICIENT" TRAINING

In most races you will want to optimize efficiency. You'll try and save your heart, and you'll try and save your legs. Or you'll try and time it so that neither one wears out before the other.

Training differs from racing. Some training time must be spent in inefficient gear selection for heart training, leg strength, and leg speed considerations.

STRENGTH TRAINING

You'll end up stronger by having "separate" workouts or aspects of workouts for leg strength or power. The legs develop more strength in bigger gears. But when you ride big gears, the intensity of your workout is not matched by your heart rate.

For example, it is not unusual for riders to train in big gears going up hills at 75% of maximum heart rate. Exertion may be similar to that perceived while riding at 85% of max heart rate in a smaller gear.

UNRELIABLE FOR ANAEROBIC WORK

Although heart-rate readings of 93% of your max and above are anaerobic, not all anaerobic efforts will result in heart rates in this range.

Your heart responds to changing exercise intensity, but this response sometimes belies actual effort. Also, monitor readings lag behind actual heart rate by several seconds. These lags mean that you may already be recovering before your monitor has the time to reflect true effort.

DON'T BE A SLAVE TO YOUR MONITOR

Riding under 65% of your max HR? You are not training your heart. But this may not be necessary.

As a case in point, recently I started training with new time-trial bars. I wanted to get used to the position. I was not training for leg strength, I was not training for leg speed. I was training for position and comfort.

I rode my easy Monday workout at an HR of 110 bpm, leg cadence of 90 rpm on rollers.

I was training, though. I was training my back muscles, my forearms, etc., and I was resting my legs, and recovering from a hard Sunday ride.

Recovering—that is an important part of training too!

CHAPTER 10

Specific Types of Training

Aerobic Training

Aerobic capacity is an important part of the training equation. The ability to use oxygen as a fuel is vital.

AEROBIC CAPACITY

Aerobic capacity is the ability to work using oxygen as a fuel to produce energy.

AEROBIC ENDURANCE

Aerobic endurance is the capacity of the body to perform aerobic work over long periods of time. This is what is important in sustained efforts—in time trialing or in long hill climbing.

To improve aerobic endurance one must improve the quantity or quality of components of this system. Aerobic endurance involves oxygen transport from the air we breathe to the chemical factories of the body that use oxygen for fuel. This includes the heart, lungs, circulation and cell transportation systems, and the cells' energy-producing mitochondria.

AEROBIC TRAINING PRINCIPLES

Aerobic training requires the rhythmic action of large muscle groups, as in cycling or running. Vigorous video game play using only smaller hand muscles can never place enough demands on the body to be aerobic.

Aerobic training begins at about 66% of an individual's maximum heart rate.

An increasing workload is required to stimulate aerobic training as an individual becomes fitter. Consequently, aerobic training should be progressive: Since the body is constantly adapting, the intensity of workouts must be increased until an individual's genetic aerobic potential is reached.

For the very fit, training at rates higher than 93% of max HR will cause anaerobic systems to kick in, allowing fewer aerobic repeats. For the less fit, anaerobic systems may take over at heart rates as low as 80% of maximum.

Besides reaching your aerobic potential, you can train to increase the length of time over which you can maintain this level of work.

Aerobic fitness may be lost in as little as 1 to 2 weeks; training regularity is important. Thirty minutes twice a week is suggested for maintenance.

INTENSITY, DURATION, FREQUENCY

To improve the aerobic system, most athletes will strive to achieve a heart rate of at least 80% of maximum for at least 30 minutes, three times per week. Endurance may be improved by training at lower levels, but maximal oxygen uptake may not increase.

Racers need 86–92% maximum heart-rate training to reach the limits of their aerobic potential. Training near this level overlaps with anaerobic training at times; this is threshold training. See table 10–1.

VALUE OF INTERVAL TRAINING

There is little proof that interval work is more helpful than continuous work at aerobic levels. There is evidence that interval training is helpful in anaerobic training. Anaerobic intervals are shorter, with maximal efforts.

Exercise pace in aerobic interval training should be similar to that of competition. Recovery intervals are designed so that many high-quality intervals can be completed in the training session.

Regular interval training may adapt the nervous system to movement patterns experienced in competition.

One may exercise longer at the limits of aerobic metabolism by performing intervals rather than by continuous training. Theoretically this may allow better physiological adaptations.

LENGTH OF THE AEROBIC INTERVAL

Aerobic intervals should be long enough to reach maximum oxygen uptake in most of the intervals, and short enough to minimize fatigue.

Because experimental results are inconclusive regarding the benefits of short (15–30 seconds) and long (up to 5 minutes) intervals for aerobic training, a variety of training intervals are recommended.

In aerobic training, short intervals require short recovery intervals—or one hasn't enough time to reach the demands of required training levels.

Mild exercise during rest intervals (heart rate 100–120 bpm) hastens recovery. Keep your legs moving!

THEORETICAL BASIS: THE OXYGEN TRANSPORT SYSTEM

Air is 21% oxygen. Air is inhaled through the nose or mouth into the lungs. As the air enters the lungs it travels down progressively smaller and smaller tubes until it reaches the air sacs, or alveoli, where oxygen is transported across fine membranes to the smallest blood vessels, the capillaries.

Entering progressively larger veins, the blood travels to the heart and is then pumped to the rest of the body, in cycling specifically the legs, where it travels down smaller and smaller arteries until it reaches the muscle capillaries where it is transported across cell membranes to muscle cells, and their energy-producing factories, the mitochondria.

ATP

In these energy factories of the cell, chemical reactions (involving adenosine triphosphate or ATP) take place that allow the production of energy. This feeds the muscle cells contracting with filaments called actin and myosin. When these filaments interact, muscle movement results.

WHAT TRAINING DOES

Adaptations to aerobic endurance training may occur in the body in any of the following ways:

- Training may help increase the amount of blood delivered to working muscles.
- Training may increase the filling of the heart in its rest phase, allowing more blood to be ejected with each heartbeat. Training may increase the strength and efficiency of the heart muscle and result in more complete emptying of the heart with each beat.
- Training may enhance the diffusion (or flow) of oxygen from capillary to muscle (because of greater stores of myoglobin).
- Training may increase the number of capillaries.
- Training may result in a greater ability of skeletal mitochondria to use oxygen, due either to greater numbers of mitochondria or to greater amounts of enzymes in each individual mitochondrion.
- Training may open up blood vessels, allowing blood to more easily reach the muscle capillaries.
- Training may shift the threshold at which work becomes anaerobic. At a given high level of work, improved training may increase the relative percentage of aerobic work. This results in less and less need for anaerobic function, which, in turn, means less lactic acid buildup.

Anaerobic Training

Anaerobic training is more important to the average racer than aerobic training. Anaerobic metabolism results in lactic acid accumulation that is poisonous to the body and prevents sustained efforts. This distinguishes aerobic metabolism from anaerobic metabolism.

ANAEROBIC POWER AND CAPACITY

Anaerobic power is the maximal rate at which energy can be produced or work can be done without a significant contribution from aerobic (mitochondrial) energy production.

Table 10-1 Aerobic Heart-Rate Guidelines

Max HR (beats per min.)	Aerobic (66–85%)	Threshold (86–92%)
205	135–174	175–189
200	132–170	171–184
195	129–166	167–179
190	125–162	163–175
185	122–157	158–170
180	119–153	154–166
175	116–149	150–161
170	112–145	146–156
165	109–140	141–152
160	106–136	137–147
155	102–132	133–143
150	99–128	129–138

Anaerobic capacity is the ability to maintain or repeat strenuous muscular contractions that rely upon anaerobic mechanisms of energy supply.

These activities can be sustained for less than 1 or 2 minutes.

Longer activities demand substantial rates of oxygen consumption and have significant aerobic components. Anaerobic power and capacity require a type of physical fitness lying between pure strength fitness and aerobic fitness. The lower anaerobic level overlaps with aerobic training and, as stated earlier, is called threshold training.

There are two main types of muscle fiber: fast twitch and slow twitch. The amount of fast- versus slow-twitch fibers in a given person is genetically predetermined.

Fast-twitch muscle fibers play a large role in anaerobic power and capacity.

A strong person who can lift a maximum weight of 48 kg might be expected to hold a weight of 16 kg twice as long as another who can lift a maximum load of only 24 kg. However, for maximum loads, both subjects might be expected to lift that weight (48 or 24 kg) for the same period of time (the stronger individual can lift a heavier weight.)

The training analogy is that stronger riders train for the same duration as weaker riders, but push bigger gears.

CYCLING AS AN ANAEROBIC SPORT

As already said, anaerobic training is more important to the average racer than aerobic training.

With the exception of time trials, competitive cycling is not a smooth, steady effort: Constant surges and changes in acceleration are required. Finishing sprints require high levels of anaerobic ability. Even pacelines require accelerations of a couple of miles per hour when tagging on to the back of the line.

The demands of racing are different from club training rides. Many new racers are surprised at the anaerobic requirements of racing, and many experienced racers are also not able to tolerate these efforts.

The ability to sustain repeated anaerobic surges requires a large anaerobic reserve capacity. The ability to recover demands a large aerobic capacity. If you train with repeated anaerobic efforts and closely spaced recovery periods, you will train both systems. Most important, you will be training in a manner very specific to the real requirements of racing.

TRAINING FOR ANAEROBIC CAPACITY MEANS ANAEROBIC INTERVALS

Exercises used to improve anaerobic capacity should mimic the actual task performance that one is attempting to improve.

Because energy for anaerobic activities is produced by anaerobic mechanisms within the body, training programs must be designed to stress these mechanisms.

It is important that training sessions produce as much high-quality work as possible. The combination of a good warm-up of 30 minutes and a cool-down of at least 15 minutes allows more high-quality work to be performed and hastens recovery.

Interval workouts contain periods of high-intensity effort, and then a recovery or rest interval in between.

This training technique allows you to perform more minutes of "supermaximal" work than you could otherwise continuously maintain. If you rode as hard as you could for as long as you could, you might ride only 1 or 2 minutes. In one early study of interval training a subject ran at a pace causing total exhaustion in less than 5 minutes and covered only 0.8 mile. Running at the same exhaustive pace, using short intervals, the subject ran for more than 20 minutes and covered 4 miles.

Figure 10–1

Interval Terms:	
Continuous	Non-interval training. Training without work and recovery periods.
Interval	A period of work, normally a relatively short, hard effort.
Recovery	Relief period between efforts.
Intensity	Load or speed of the work or resistance to overcome.
Repetitions	Number of efforts undertaken within a set or training session.
Duration	Length of a period of specified work/interval without rest.
Volume	The total time of intense work. If training is continuous, volume and duration are the same.

Exercise physiologists and sports scientists use interval terms to describe work and rest periods. Cyclists employ the word *interval* more narrowly, normally referring to efforts lasting between 1 and 6 minutes. More information about cycling interval workouts is found later in this chapter.

LENGTH OF THE WORK INTERVAL

Anaerobic power intervals must last no longer than a few minutes. Work intervals longer than this duration rely too much on aerobic energy production.

The total time spent performing high-quality work intervals is normally 10 to 20 minutes. It is reasonable to start with a total of just 3 to 5 minutes of high-quality anaerobic interval work.

INTENSITY OF THE WORK INTERVAL

The speed should be similar to or faster than your training goal. For example, if you are trying to achieve a 4-minute pursuit time for 3,000 meters, then 500-meter times must be faster than 40 seconds.

Have a specific workout goal in mind. Your schedule might allow some flexibility, but do not simply ride hard for "as long as you feel like it" and see how you do. Decide on your program, have a set goal of, say, ten 15-second intervals on Tuesdays and five 60-second and five 90-second intervals on Thursdays, and try to stick to it.

When you are tired you should maintain the speed/quality of the intervals but reduce the number of repetitions.

Work intervals shorter than 20 seconds do not bring about maximal amounts of anaerobic energy production unless combined with recovery intervals of less than 30 seconds. Otherwise too much aerobic ATP replenishment occurs during recovery intervals.

Intensity must be maximal or nearly maximal. At least 90% of maximal effort is recommended. For intervals of less than 30 seconds you ride absolutely all-out as hard as you can. For longer efforts you ride as hard as you can to make the time. If you can't make the time, back off a little.

For intervals of less than 60 seconds, heart-rate monitoring is unreliable: The effort will be done before your heart rate "catches up." For longer efforts, your heart rate should be close to or above your threshold. See table 10–2.

RECOVERY INTERVAL

Recovery intervals must be long enough to allow substantial recovery of muscles but short enough to continue and increase stress. Recovery intervals following short work intervals (20–30 seconds) should be up to 2 minutes. Longer work intervals of 1 to 2 minutes may require more complete recovery periods.

Lactic acid is removed from muscles more rapidly when mild exercise,

Table 10–2 **Anaerobic Heart-Rate Guidelines**

Max HR (beats per min.)	Threshold (86–92%)	Anaerobic (93+%)
205	175–189	190
200	171–184	185
195	167–179	180
190	163–175	176
185	158–170	171
180	154–166	167
175	150–161	162
170	146–156	157
165	141–152	153
160	137–147	148
155	133–143	144
150	129–138	139

rather than complete inactivity, is performed during recovery, so easy cycling between work intervals is recommended.

FREQUENCY OF SESSIONS

For pure anaerobic training, in non-cycling sports, three to four sessions per week may be optimal. To allow for a rounding out of cycling needs such as endurance, and considering that race weekends are taxing efforts, one or two specific interval sessions per week is a reasonable number.

Many combinations of work and recovery intervals can be used. You can, for example, perform several sets of intervals of different durations, with more complete recovery between sets.

It is important to vary the approach to anaerobic training so that boredom does not cause you to drop the training program.

The result of anaerobic interval training is improved anaerobic and aerobic capacity.

The same work interval combined with different recovery intervals may be used to specifically train for different cycling events. For example, 10-second all-out work intervals (sprints) with 5-minute recovery intervals might be used

Table 10-3 **Suggested Schemes for Anaerobic Interval Training**

Work Interval Duration	Effort Intensity %	Recovery Interval (length)	Work Intervals/ Session	Sessions per Week
10 sec	100	10+ sec	20–30	2
20 sec	100	20+ sec	10–20	2
30 sec	98+	1–2 min	8–18	2
60 sec	95+	3–5 min	5–15	2
90 sec	92+	3–10 min	5–12	2
2 min	90+	5–15 min	4–10	2

to train track sprinting. Ten-second work intervals with 10-second recovery intervals might be used to train criterium demands.

Effort intensity refers to perceived effort: 100% effort means you work absolutely as hard as you can. Since efforts are short, heart rate will not have enough time to "catch up" and you must rely on perceived exertion rather than on any objective heart-rate measurement—you work as hard as you can just to be able to complete the interval.

Interval Training

WHAT ARE INTERVALS?

Cyclists use the word *interval* to specifically denote training at intensities below those found in sprints and above those in a 10-mile time trial. Exercise physiologists include sprints in their definition of intervals. Cyclists don't.

Exercise physiologists use the word *interval* to denote *any* work period. So intervals can be aerobic if done below threshold intensity or anaerobic if performed above this level. Anaerobic intervals and the physiologic point of view were discussed more fully earlier in this chapter.

It's not that one definition is right or wrong, it's just cycling jargon vs. science jargon.

Cycling interval training differs from sprint work in several respects: Sprints are faster and shorter. More time is allowed for recovery between work periods in sprints, often with a slower pace between work periods.

INTERVAL TRAINING WORKS

The benefits of interval training include improved acceleration, high-speed endurance, and the ability to respond to a changing pace. Interval training is a relative shortcut to improving speed and strength. It has proven to help anaerobic power and capacity.

EXAMPLES OF INTERVALS

Assume you can ride a time trial at 24 miles an hour for 10 miles. Interval work might consist of 5 to 10 hard 1-mile efforts at 26+ mph.

Another technique is decreasing intervals. For example, you might ride as hard as you can maintain for 2 minutes, and then ride each successive interval for 10 fewer seconds, down to 30 to 60 seconds.

Another type of interval is the hill interval. Distances of 0.5 to 1.5 miles up a steady grade might be used. On a 1-mile climb you might ride as fast as possible up the 1-mile climb, coast down to recover, and then repeat another 5 times.

HEART-RATE MONITOR?

A heart-rate monitor can be very helpful in assuring that you are making a hard effort during intervals. Many inexperienced riders benefit from the feedback that heart-rate monitors provide. Many experienced racers like to confirm their intensity. Most coaches swear by their value.

Remember, for short intervals, or intervals not preceded by a good warm-up or high-aerobic level of work, heart rate might not "catch up" to effort.

U.S. multiple time-trial record holder Jane Gagne has another point of view. She doesn't see the need for heart-rate monitoring: "Basically you ride as hard as you can to complete the interval—it doesn't matter what your heart rate is."

HOW OFTEN?

Cycling interval work is done *formally* once or twice a week. Race day also provides interval work. Interval workouts may be your hardest training day.

Since time is needed to recover before race day, most coaches suggest intervals be done at least 3 days before race day.

Leg-Speed Work

The ability to turn the legs quickly is crucial in sprinting and surging. This neuromuscular skill—independent of strength and aerobic and anaerobic capacity—is a vital aspect of fitness for the all-round racer.

WHAT WE'RE TALKING ABOUT

The ability to move the legs fast. We're talking about a couple of types of leg speed: the ability to turn extremely rapidly for very short periods of time and the ability to maintain a relatively high cadence for longer periods.

Recreational riders often move their legs with a cadence of about 70 revolutions per minute. Typically, time trialists have a cadence of 85 rpm, road riders 95 rpm, and crit riders 100+ rpm. Sprints may be well over 150 rpm, with track sprinters having the ability to turn their cranks at over 250 rpm on trainers for brief periods.

Think about driving a five-speed stick-shift car down a curvy country road. At 50 mph, the best fuel economy will be in fifth gear. If you want to pass a car, you'll get more jump by down-shifting to fourth.

Steady riding at slow speeds is easier at lower cadences. But surges, jumps, and sprints are much more effective at faster cadence.

HOW TO GET LEG SPEED

How else? Like everything else! With practice.

FITTING THE WORKOUTS IN

Leg-speed workouts are done in very easy to moderate gears. They emphasize leg speed, not leg power or cardiovascular capacity. In that sense they are not fatiguing. They can be performed on recovery days or incorporated into longer workouts that train other aspects of fitness.

Figure 10–2 **Leg-speed workout #1: improving overall leg speed.**

Very easy gear.

- Warm-up: Start at 60 rpm. Increase by 5 rpm every minute until you're spinning at 120 rpm.
- Rest a few minutes.
- Start at 80 rpm. Increase by 5 rpm every minute until at 130 rpm.
- Rest a few minutes.
- Start at 80 rpm. Increase by 5 rpm every 30 seconds until you're spun out.

Aim for 140 rpm by the end of your first season.
Aim for 150 rpm by the end of your second season.

Figure 10–3 **Leg-speed workout #2: sustaining leg speed.**

Very easy gear.

- Warm-up: Start at 60 rpm. Increase by 5 rpm every minute until you're spinning at 120 rpm.
- Rest a few minutes.
- Spin at least 110 rpm for 10 minutes.

Aim for 110 rpm by the end of your first month of training.
Aim for 120 rpm by the end of your first season.
Aim for 125 rpm by the end of your second season.

Figure 10–4 **Leg-speed workout #3: developing peak leg speed.**

Moderate gear.

- Warm-up: Start at 60 rpm. Increase by 5 rpm every minute until you're spinning at 120 rpm.
- Rest a few minutes.
- Sprint as hard as you can, spinning as fast as you can for 15–20 seconds.

You should be spun out at the end of the interval.

Aim for 150+ rpm at the end of your first season.
Aim for 165+ rpm at the end of your second season.

Leg Strength and Power Work

The ability to produce muscular leg force is vital for all racers. Leg strength—independent of aerobic and anaerobic capacity—can be specifically trained.

WHAT WE'RE TALKING ABOUT

The ability to produce muscular force in the legs. Strictly speaking, strength refers to the maximum force that can be generated in a single maximal effort, and power refers to force over time. The two are closely related.

PHYSIOLOGY A FACTOR

Power is related to the size of muscle fibers, the percentage of muscle fibers activated at any one time, muscle-cell energy production, blood supply, lactic acid metabolism, and muscular economy.

WEIGHT-LIFTING ANALOGY

In order to develop strength, many athletes go to the gym. A weight lifter might have the option of lifting 50 pounds 30 times, lifting 75 pounds 20 times, or lifting 100 pounds 8 times.

Lifting the heavier weight will result in greater strength gains. Lifting the lighter weight is associated with less injury and more general conditioning.

CYCLING MESSAGE

In order to develop strength and power, workouts that emphasize heavy gears with high loads and low rpm result in more strength gains than more moderate loads with higher rpm.

Strength and power workouts should not be performed until general conditioning has taken place.

Figure 10-5 **Leg strength workout #1.**

- Push the heaviest gear you can for 15 minutes at 50 rpm and at a heart rate of about 75% of your max.
- Rest for 5 minutes.
- Repeat one or two times.

If performed on the road, most riders find this workout best on steady climbs of about 5% grade. Fifteen minutes usually means a climb of about 3 miles.

If you wish to work on hill muscle strength, climb with your hands on the tops.

If you wish to work on time trialing or flat land strength, climb in the drops.

If you perform this workout correctly, you'll notice that you could go faster in an easier gear. But the point of the workout is not maximizing overall speed, it's maximizing strength.

Figure 10-6 **Leg strength workout #2: isolated leg training.**

One-legged riding builds strength and smoothness.

- Unclip your right foot from the right pedal. Ride at 50 rpm with just your left leg in as hard a gear as you can maintain for 3-5 minutes.
- Rest for a couple of minutes, riding with both legs. Alternate and ride with the right leg for 3–5 minutes.
- Rest 5 minutes.
- Repeat one or two times.

Sprintwork

A good sprint is needed to finish well at the end of a race.

Bursts of speed are also required at many other times. If primes (prizes) are given for winners of individual laps on a circuit course, you'll need that sprint.

If several riders are up ahead and you want to catch up, you'll need a good jump to be able to catch them alone. (Catching them, with everyone else behind you, is not jumping or sprinting, it is pulling.)

SPRINTING COMPONENTS

To sprint well in a race you need:

- Good jump power.
- Good leg speed.

- Good tactics.
- Good technique—physical and mental.

Practicing jumps is crucial. A good jump comes from power. Weight training is valuable for strength and power training. Bicycle-specific strength work, including big-gear riding and isolated leg training, was described earlier in this chapter.

Leg speed is developed by training in an easy gear and was discussed earlier in this chapter. Fixed-gear training can help.

Tactics come from exercises in small- and large-group practice, and from race experience.

The physical technique of sprinting involves placing the hands in the drops, proper distribution of body weight to prevent skidding or wheelies, and changing pedal emphasis from sudden downward strokes to a smooth spin.

The mental technique requires a psychological readjustment from hard, steady-state riding to the sharp, total commitment of pure anaerobic effort. Lack of mental force inhibits many riders who have the physical ability to do better.

SPRINTING VS. SPEEDWORK

Sprinting is making the bike go fast. Speedwork is making the legs go fast. They are not the same thing. Sprinting is the marriage of power and leg speed.

SPRINT WORKOUTS

Sprint workouts consist of hard jumps, all-out efforts to go as fast as you can. You go as hard as you possibly can for 10 to 20 seconds.

PHASES OF A SPRINT

The sprint can be divided into three phases:

- The jump, or initial acceleration.
- The spin section at speed.
- The final kick or holding on to the finish.

To jump, you get out of your saddle, sprinting to near maximum rpm. Then sit down and hold that top speed for the distance. Most riders slightly increase their rpm while sitting.

GEARING

What gears you use depends upon the terrain, wind, and your condition. You can accelerate more quickly in an easier gear. It's like accelerating a stick-shift car—you often can jump faster by using an easier gear.

If you start your sprint from a relatively low speed, you'll probably practice sprints in the big chain ring with about a 17-tooth cog. You may need to shift to a bigger gear when you sit down.

If you start your sprint from a relatively high speed, you may use a bigger gear.

Sprintwork in small gears emphasizes leg speed. Sprintwork in big gears emphasizes strength and power.

PRACTICE SPRINTS WHEN FRESH

Sprints in practice are different from sprints in races. With sprint practice you are working on this specific aspect of racing only. In a race, you may already be tired and your sprint may be poor.

Sprint training when you are fresh allows you to improve your leg speed and jump. It allows you to selectively train the specific components needed to sprint well.

Occasionally, to simulate races, you may wish to sprint at the end of training rides when you are tired.

GIVE SPRINTS 100% EFFORT

When you practice sprintwork, and you want to "do it right," you ride with all your heart, your 100% maximum effort. This will make you stronger and faster.

RECOVERY PERIOD

After a hard sprint you are tired. Immediately shift to an easy gear, spin easily, ride slowly, relax. It may take more than 5 minutes to feel recovered. Then go again.

HOW MANY REPETITIONS?

On a sprint day practice, do at least 6 sprints, but never as many as 15. If you can do 15, you have not worked as hard as you could have on the earlier sprints in your practice.

GROUP PRACTICE

With a group of riders you can practice sprints side by side with agreed-upon gears. Avoid practicing sprint tactics exclusively. If you do, tactics will play too much of a part in your practice, and you won't be training your anaerobic system to its potential.

Once good-quality speedwork training is part of your week, you can practice sprints with a group simulating race conditions.

- You can practice sprinting with a leadout. This is riding behind another rider who is willing to push hard well before the finish line in order to pull you up and allow you to sprint for the finish yourself. This is an important aspect of team tactics at the end of the race, when the person giving the leadout is your teammate and does so willingly. It is also an important race strategy when you glue up behind a fast rider who does it for you less than willingly.
- You can practice with a small group, positioning yourself and sprinting for an agreed-upon finish line.

Fixed-Gear Training

Fixed-gear bicycles have no choice in gearing. Fixed-gear training gives you leg strength and leg speed. Good training all year round, it is especially helpful in the off-season.

FIXED-GEAR BIKES DEFINED

A fixed-gear road bike is one with no choice of gears. As the bike moves so must your legs. You are forced to pedal. This helps develop a smooth pedal stroke. You can't shift when climbing hills—this helps develop power. You can't shift when going down hills—this helps your leg speed. You can't stop pedaling going around corners—this helps cornering skills. As you fly down hills, after a few weeks of fixed-gear riding, you may be able to spin at 200+ rpm. The fast and slow pedaling that fixed-gear riding demands will give your legs an important range of rpm ability.

CREATE A FIXED-GEAR BIKE

If you have a track bike you need to add (at least) a front brake.
  On your road bike with horizontal dropouts:

- You can substitute a single cog (narrow pitch for your road chain) for your freewheel with a bottom bracket ring as a lock ring.
- You can solder/weld/glue shut a freewheel.
- You can use a track rear wheel on your road bike. This has the advantage of a more solid hub that stands up better to the torque of fixed-gear riding. On a track hub you can thread a road cog, or use a track cog with a track chain on your road chain ring.
- You can take off your derailleurs. If you leave your rear derailleur on, you must omit threading the jockey pulleys. You must shorten your chain. You may need to use spacers to get the chain correctly aligned.

WHAT GEAR?

You might try using the small chain ring in front and a 15-cog to start.

EARLY PRACTICE

Start with short rides on the level. Avoid major descents and tight corners. Use your brakes to keep you from spinning out of control and going over your handlebars when going down inclines. Back pedaling may also slow your speed. As you learn to spin and to corner, you'll be able to safely handle steeper descents and tighter corners.

Training with a Weaker Rider

Riders of quite different abilities can easily train together. Flexibility in training method and an honest regard for the weaker rider are required.

WHY TRAIN WITH A WEAKER RIDER?

My wife, Gero, and I share many things in common. We both love riding bicycles, we are both somewhat competitive, and we both love each other. We're both pretty good riders. But we are also very different.

She could ride a 10-mile trial in about 30 minutes—the last one she actually rode was about 6 years ago. She can't remember why in heaven's name she did it! I ride more than 8 minutes faster than that. She's definitely not a racer, and I place with the Category 1, 2's.

I know quite a few other racers, but few ride with their "significant others"—girlfriends or wives. That seems to me a pity because, after all, the reason Gero is my wife is that I do like to be with her.

Judging by her and others' comments, many of the women she rides with would like to ride with their partners, if their partners wouldn't always leave them in the dust.

There are ways to ride with a weaker rider so that both of you get everything you want and need out of a ride. Let me share a few hints. After a while I am sure you will be able to come up with even more suggestions on your own.

RESPECT THE NEEDS OF THE WEAKER RIDER

If you are truly riding with a weaker rider, don't try to beat her up. There is no point in trying to show you are a superior rider and being competitive with someone you care about. If someone wins, someone loses. And if you are talking about riding with someone close to you, you lose. This seems to me to be less of a problem with parents and kids. Parents seem to be a lot more protective of their kids than of their spouses or friends. As soon as you realize that riding with a weaker rider means not having to prove how strong you are, you can start having fun.

AGREE ON RIDE EXPECTATIONS

The next generalization is that you must have reasonable expectations for the ride. If you want to ride 100 miles in 4 hours, and your weaker partner can manage 40 miles in 3 hours, don't ride together that day.

If you want to practice pack skills in a tight group to simulate criterium riding, don't look to your pack-shy friend to help you out on that one. If you want most other things, most of the time you can get them. You can get speed, strength, and intensity. You may be able to get bike-handling skills.

It is helpful, though, if your weaker partner realizes that what you are doing is meant to help both of you. It helps to enlist your partner to help you improve. Of course the weaker rider may improve too, but that is requisite only if the rider wants to.

TRAINING EXAMPLES

Let me give you some examples: Two years ago I went on a lovely 10-day ride through southeastern California with my wife. We traveled 700 miles, which was the distance both of us desired. So we were on the same wavelength. But if I rode at her speed the whole time, I felt I would lose fitness. So for a lark, I decided to ride the whole ride in a 42/15. Right away this prevented me from going too fast for her. It forced me to work like the dickens going up steep hills and mountains. It forced me to work like crazy to catch back up on descents. On the flats I was mostly happy to rest and recover. So it worked wonders for strength on the uphills, and was fantastic for leg speed trying to keep up and draft her on slight downhills. It was great for Gero because she could, at times, outrun me, and make me hurt. (And sometimes she likes doing that.) Most days we finished equally pooped.

When Gero and I climb hills together there are any number of ways we stay pretty close together on the climb. And, of course, it is usually on hills that the stronger rider just floats away leaving the weaker rider alone.

Perhaps the strongest I have ever been as a hill climber was one of the first seasons I raced, in 1986. Gero and I would ride each Saturday, about 15 miles someplace for lunch, and 15 miles back. Sunday I rode with the fast boys in the Banana Gang.

The technique that made me so strong was that I sat upright on the bike, and pushed Gero up the hills. Find the right gear, usually the biggest one you can comfortably push, place your hand flat on the back of your partner, and push steadily. Give your partner and yourself a break every once in a while, and stand and stretch.

Sure I could have gone faster myself, but I doubt I would have become stronger. Gero, not wanting to let me down, became very strong. And I, not wanting to let her down, pushed even harder. It was great!

Last year I worked on time trialing. Gero and I climbed 4,000 feet in 16 miles to a local mountaintop. The first 8 miles I stood in a big gear, at about 30 rpm, never sitting down. I went at Gero's pace. In some ways it is even harder to go more slowly in a big gear. It builds tremendous leg strength. Try it some time.

For the next few miles I relaxed at Gero's pace, and pushed her some of the way. For the last 5 miles I climbed seated, with my hands in the drops, in a big gear at about 40 rpm, a terribly inefficient way to climb. Power falls when riding in the drops because your muscles' maximum forces cannot be applied. Riding in the drops would be an inefficient way to ride on the flats as well, were it not for wind drag.

But here's a secret. Sometimes training inefficiently in one setting increases efficiency in another. Climbing in the drops may not make you a better climber, but it will make you a better time trialist, because that is how you time-trial, and climbing that way gets to those time-trial muscle groups and makes them strong. I'd never climb that way in a race, I'd be dropped. Behind my wife, I can go at just that right speed so that *she* leads *me* up the climb.

Another day, on another trip, I rode intervals behind my wife all day. Behind? You bet. I was allowed to ride with only one leg at a time. This technique gave strength, improved my pedal stroke, and made her feel like a million dollars every time we sprinted for a city limit sign and she beat me! Of course, you can do regular intervals too, for the innumerable milepost signs and city limit signs, or just by watching your bike computer. If you just make one small circle back, and ride slowly to recover after such an interval, your partner will be there in no time. Don't leave your partner too long in case there has been a flat or other accident.

TANDEM POSSIBILITIES

For several summers Gero and I toured on a tandem. One summer we toured Colorado, climbing to over 12,000 feet on Independence Pass. The secret to tandem riding is not to surprise your partner and to communicate frequently about gear shifts, stops, etc. Each partner works as hard as he or she wants. You do have to agree on cadence and speed on descents. On climbs one or both can stand at a time. The stronger rider can stand for longer periods. The captain (lead rider) has to give the stoker a chance periodically to stretch and get off the seat—on a single bike you can do this whenever you like, but on a tandem you have to coordinate.

Nelson Cronyn has his wife, Judith, unclip, then perform "sprints" of about 50 pedal revolutions. He finds this great for leg strength.

In 1992 I set the Masters 40K Tandem Time Trial Record (46:45) with Jerry Logan at Moriarty, New Mexico. Jerry flew back to San Diego, while I toured New Mexico with Gero. I rode the tandem, with rack and panniers added, alone. Gero rode her single, unencumbered. With the tandem and bags weighing about 75 pounds, it wasn't so easy to get to the mountaintops first!

HELP YOUR PARTNER DRAFT

Teaching your partner to draft effectively is another way to increase your collective speed. Don't teach your partner this technique at too fast a pace— your partner will be so frightened by the pace that he or she will not be able to concentrate on the technique. When you do draft, check frequently with your partner to make sure the pace is okay, and try to avoid burning them off the back. Let your partner lead occasionally too—your partner will learn how to lead better, and you can practice technique, ride with one leg, or just rest.

TEACH YOUR PARTNER SKILLS

Bike-handling skills? Most of the guys I know think their wives are not interested in bike-handling skills because they never seem to want to get close, fall down, ride in a big group, or shove. I've got news for you. In a controlled, safe way, almost everybody loves proximity drills and bike-handling games. With just me in the grassy park nearby, Gero thrills at trying to pick a water bottle off the ground, or practicing touching wheels. It's when the danger is beyond control that we may get afraid. Teach your friends these skills. They will appreciate them. Another little secret: When you teach people about something, you learn more yourself.

ENJOY YOUR PARTNER'S COMPANY

There are a million games you can play. You can train with a weaker rider. I love to race, I love to ride with the fast boys on the Banana Gang. And I love to ride with Gero.

Stretching

WHY STRETCH?

Stretching helps increase flexibility. Joint motion is limited by joint capsules, ligaments, and muscles. These tissues can be successfully stretched with exercises. Some stretching merely has a temporary effect, based on the elastic properties of the tissue stretched. Other effects of stretching can be long-lasting.

Stretches are obviously important in athletic efforts such as gymnastics. Stretching may also help to prevent injuries and strains. Whether increased flexibility results in improved performance in bicycling is subject to some debate. Most coaches and bicyclists who stretch believe it is helpful. Hard "scientific" data are lacking.

GUIDELINES

- A stretch workout can be done in 15 minutes. If you have the time it can easily occupy a half hour.
- Develop a stretching routine, and perform your stretches in the same order. Such a routine helps you to perform all your stretches and not miss any.
- Some joints can be stretched in several directions. Develop your routine so as to stretch these complementary motions in sequence. For example, after arching your back, as in Figure 10–10, bend it forward, as in Figure 10–11.
- Stretch slowly and gradually. Avoid bouncing or ballistic motions. There is a basic neurologic reflex called the "stretch reflex." When a muscle is suddenly stretched, the reflex contracts or shortens the muscle. If you stretch slowly the reflex is not activated. Fast stretching is counterproductive.
- Stretch to tightness, but not to the point of pain.

- Hold stretches for at least 20 and up to 60 seconds.
- Stretching is more effective when the muscles are warm, not cold. Avoid stretching first thing in the morning when you are otherwise stiff. If your routine provides the time to stretch in the morning, first ride your trainer easily for 10 minutes, or do some other general exercise. Stretching is probably more helpful after a bicycle ride than before one.

Figure 10–7

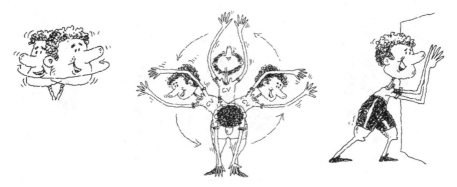

Figure 10–8

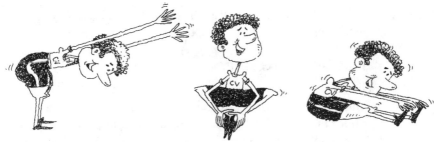

Figure 10–9

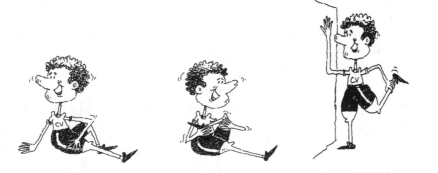

Figure 10–10

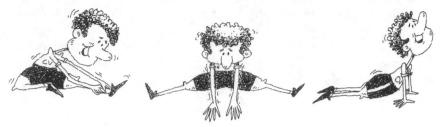

Figure 10–10

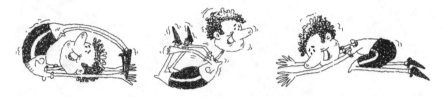

Figure 10–11

Weight Training

WHY LIFT WEIGHTS?

The number-one reason dedicated cyclists lift weights is because they believe it will make their muscles stronger and more powerful and thereby improve their cycling.

Lifting weights has a number of other benefits:

• Weight training helps develop overall body strength. It helps develop upper-body strength for bicycle control, leverage in climbing, and improved chest expansion. It can help strengthen back and stomach muscles and may help reduce back problems.
• Weight training helps correct imbalances and improve postural changes from cycling.
• Weight training helps achieve symmetrical right- and left-sided strength.
• Weight training helps balance agonist/antagonist muscles—that is, push/pull or flexion/extension muscles.

While most cycling coaches endorse weight work, not all believe it is important—especially for elite road riders. Weight work may be most important for cyclists in the first few years of their cycling careers to build leg strength.

Bicycling is the most specific form of exercise for the cyclist. Bicycling strength work with isolated leg training or big-gear work at low cadence is more specific than weight work. Many riders notice that weight training detracts from their climbing ability.

Track sprinters may be a special breed. Their specific need for fast-twitch muscle fiber strength almost demands weight work. It may be vital for developing explosive strength and power for legs.

Almost every year there are articles in the national magazines about the weight work that the top U.S. sprinter performs. On the other hand, Vic Copeland, who set more track records than any rider in U.S. history and revolutionized the concept of fast-twitch masters riders, never lifted weights.

CAUTION!

You are a bicycle rider, not a weight lifter. Your most important lifting priority is not to be injured lifting. About one-half the racers I know who lift weights injure themselves while lifting.

There are proper techniques in lifting. Ideally, you'll want to be instructed in proper form to prevent injury.

It's common for muscles to strengthen faster than supporting tendons and ligaments. Even though your muscles may be ready for more work, the rest of you may not be. If you are an older rider, it is common for degenerative joint disease related to aging—osteoarthritis—to limit your ability to safely lift very heavy weights.

It takes years for the body to adapt to lifting. It's easy to injure yourself by attempting to lift more than your body is ready to lift.

LIFTING HINTS

- Comfortable clothes make the workout easier.
- Cycling gloves help give a better grip.
- Shoes should be comfortable and supportive.
- If you have the time, warm up with light calisthenics, stretching, and a light exercise set. This helps prevent injuries.
- Develop a routine and go from exercise to exercise, wasting little time. But have enough of a rest between sets so that your heart rate recovers completely.
- Try to be efficient, allowing your workout to take about 1 hour.
- Work large muscle groups before small ones.
- Work first the muscle groups that are most important to you. That way if you are interrupted or have limited time, you'll be sure to have done the most important exercises.
- Increase weights gradually and steadily.
- Remember to breathe. Breathe out during the power or lifting phase, breathe in during the relaxation phase.
- Always use collars on adjustable free weights.

WHEN?

Weight training makes the most sense in the off-season, from October to February/March.

Track riders may weight-train year-round.

HOW OFTEN?

Most riders lift two or three times a week. If winter means snow and you are not riding much, three times a week will allow more gains than twice a week.

If you continue to ride, I suggest lifting twice a week. In addition to lifting, perform a strength ride or two each week with big-gear climbs or isolated-leg training. Don't forget to spend a considerable portion of the rest of your week spinning.

REPETITIONS AND SETS

Repetitions are the number of times in a row you perform an exercise. Groups of reps are called a set. For example, doing an exercise 12 times, resting, then going again is 2 sets of 12 reps.

COACHING PHILOSOPHY

The most important decision is whether to begin lifting. Coaches disagree as to how many reps and how many sets are optimal for bicyclists. Most cycling authorities say you should do 6–20 reps of each exercise in your set. Some advocate up to 50 reps. Seasoned track sprinters may rep as few as 3–6 times.

I believe an appropriately weighted 15-rep single set provides most of the gain.

In general, you'll use fewer reps for larger muscle groups and more reps for smaller muscle groups. You might perform 12 squats and 75 sit-ups—it's rarely the other way around.

When you lift a weight that allows you to perform at least 15 reps, you strengthen both fast- and slow-twitch muscle fibers. This is most helpful for the all-round rider.

If you lift heavier weights that can only be lifted a few times, you hypertrophy (enlarge) fast-twitch muscle fibers selectively. This may result in increased explosive strength and benefit sprinting, but the increased size of these fibers relative to the overall muscle may slow down your hill climbing.

Performing more than 40 or 50 repetitions of any exercise gets time-consuming and boring. Increase the resistance before you reach this point.

Body builders often perform 5 sets of each exercise and spend hours each day in the gym. You'll hear about strength and conditioning coaches who will have athletes perform sets of 2–6 reps for maximum strength and power.

I believe that a single, well-performed set provides most of the gain. After that, returns are present, but diminished.

HOW MUCH SHOULD YOU LIFT?

Traditional strength and conditioning coaches determine how much you should lift based on percentages of the maximum amount you can lift once—the 1-rep maximum. In order to determine the maximum amount you can lift you must add progressively more weight until you fail to perform the exercise. While this method has its value for athletes in sports that demand precision in high-weight low-rep sets, I believe it is inappropriate for all but sprinters who have lifted for several seasons.

I believe it is safer and more appropriate for most cyclists to determine the weight to lift by trial and error, finding an amount that can be lifted 15 times. As training phases progress, weight can be added when the number of reps performed exceeds a nominal number, for example, 18 reps.

I have a different philosophy than many strength and conditioning coaches. Sports such as Olympic-style weight lifting, boxing, and football require explosive maximum power. But cycling usually isn't that kind of sport. It's much more aerobic. Although, with proper technique, lifting very heavy weights may not be dangerous, many cyclists just don't spend the time to learn the proper techniques. For these and other reasons I suggest that for your first two seasons of lifting you lift no more than the weight that you can rep 10 times, about 50–70% of the maximum you can lift once.

Lifting closer to maximum weight possible (for fewer reps) results in more bulk and improved sprinting, but slower climbing and less endurance. If you are a track sprinter and have been lifting for two or more years, and are properly coached in lifting techniques, it may be reasonable to lift more than 50–70% of maximum.

Lifting closer to your max makes the use of a spotter essential for many exercises.

A possible goal is to do large-muscle, upper-extremity exercises at half body weight. Big-muscle leg exercises can be done at body weight. As you start doing squats at weights beyond your body weight, back strain becomes more of a risk. Machines or other exercises, such as step-ups, may provide an alternative.

RESIDUAL ASPECT OF STRENGTH

Although it takes years to adapt to heavy weight work, it takes much less time to return to strength training if you've lifted before. There is a considerable residual aspect of strength. For example, in my third season of lifting it took me just 1 month to achieve what had taken 5 months in my first winter of weight training.

CIRCUIT TRAINING

Circuit training is weight training in which the rest intervals between different exercises are short. An attempt is made to combine weight training with cardiovascular benefit and heart rates in the aerobic training range. Circuit training is similar to the program I advocate in that weights rarely exceed the 50–70%-of-one-rep maximum and about 15 reps are performed at each station.

If you are still performing aerobic training with road bike, mountain bike, cyclocross, or stationary bicycle, or cross-training such as cross-country skiing, I see little need to mix in a cardiovascular workout in the weight room and reduce the focus you could have on strength work.

PERIODIZATION

Weight lifting fits into the strength development period of the cyclist's training year. Weight lifting itself is periodized. Consider the following periods:

TRANSITION TO WEIGHT LIFTING—NOVEMBER

By going easy the first few weeks you'll go a long way in preventing the muscle soreness that is so common when a weight program is first begun.

- Spend 2 or 3 weeks learning the machines or the exercises you have decided to perform.
- Establish your workout routine, the order in which you will perform the exercises.
- Get used to weight training gradually, lifting 15–20 reps at weights that you could easily rep 25.

STRENGTH HYPERTROPHY—END OF NOVEMBER TO MID-DECEMBER

Spend 2 or 3 weeks gradually increasing the weights to a level at which you can just rep 15–20 times and you can't lift more. When you can perform more than 18 to 20 reps, increase the weight about 10 pounds for large muscle groups and 5 pounds for smaller muscle groups.

Now you know each exercise well. If you lifted 18 reps at a certain weight 2 days ago, you know that 19 or 20 might be possible, but 25 is too much.

POWER PERIOD—MID-DECEMBER TO MID-FEBRUARY

If this is your first or second year of lifting, continue to work on strength. Each set is to max reps. If you perform 18 reps it is because you worked hard and couldn't make 19. If someone comes up to you while you are near the end of your set and begins to chat, the distraction may prevent you from finishing the exercise. Each set takes concentration.

When you are an experienced lifter, first perform a warm-up set, or a few reps at slow or moderate speed. Then perform the remaining reps with speed. You may decrease the amount you lift by about 10%.

I define strength and power training somewhat differently than do strength and conditioning coaches. In order to develop maximum possible strength and power, S&C coaches increase the weight and reduce the reps. But unless you are an elite track racer, that's not our goal. We are always aiming for about 15 reps.

TRANSITION TO CYCLING INTERVALS—MID-FEBRUARY TO MARCH

Cut back on your weight training and concentrate more on interval work on your bike. Perhaps you will do one set of each exercise twice a week instead of two or three sets three times a week. This taper may take a month.

EXERCISES

There are hundreds of exercises you can perform. Weight-training books or gym staff can assist you in choosing appropriate exercises. The most important muscle groups you'll want to work on are:

- Quads—the main bicycling-muscle group at the front of the thigh.
- Gluts—the buttocks muscles vital in high-power-output riding (time trialing and climbing).
- Triceps—muscles at the back of the arms between the elbow and shoulder, they're what you use when riding in the drops to hold yourself in the aero position.
- Back—sometimes recruited in climbing; a weak muscle group in most cyclists, and often a source of pain.
- Abdominals—also relatively weak in most riders; strength here helps reduce back pain.

My favorite exercises are below. They are not all-inclusive. They are a starting point. Most can be done with an inexpensive home gym. You'll need a couple of barbells, about 200 pounds of weights, and a bench with leg-extension and leg-curl bars. If you have access to a gym, the leg presses, pull-ups, and dips are important additions to the lifting routine. Push-ups require no equipment and are also useful.

In the early-November-transition-to-weight-training period, determine which machines or exercises you like. You'll probably want at least two for your quads and one for each of your other major leg-muscle groups. Squats are the most commonly prescribed bicycling weight-room exercise because they are often good for cyclists. Leg extensions are perhaps the most commonly performed because leg-extension machines are so readily available. But leg extensions—although a good exercise—are not as bicycling specific, and can worsen knee problems for those with condromalacia or patello-femoral dysfunction.

Step-ups a Favorite

My favorite exercise is step-ups. The muscles used are the most important ones in bicycling. Since you are using just one leg, the weight can be about a third of that used for squats. With less weight, you may not need a squat rack or spotter, and back strain can be reduced.

Figure 10–12

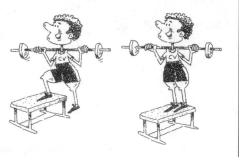

STEP-UPS: upper thighs. Perform with barbell on the back or hand-held weights. With one leg, raise up on a bench or steps to about 16 inches. Lower and repeat with the same leg for a total of 15–20 repetitions. Then use other leg.

Leg Pulls Are a Secret Weapon!

Hip-flexor strength helps you pull up during the pedal stroke. To perform this exercise, co-opt a leg curl machine.

Figure 10–13

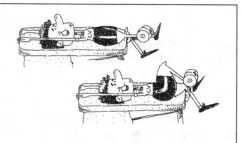

LEG PULLS: hip flexors. Use the leg curl machine, but lie on back, not prone. Hook one foot under the bar, and pull leg up toward chest. Using both legs at once makes this more of an abdominal exercise.

Other Leg Exercises

Figure 10–14

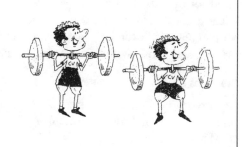

SQUATS: thighs and buttocks. Feet shoulder width apart, head up, back flat, not rounded. Full squats are to the point that your thighs are parallel to the ground. Half squats, to a lesser distance, reduce the risk of injury and are preferred, especially for first-year lifters.

Figure 10–15

LEG PRESS: upper thighs.
Adjust chair position so that in
contracted position knee position
is similar to maximum bend in
cycling. Reducing the degree of
knee flexion when contracted
reduces the risk of injury. Press
out until legs almost extended.

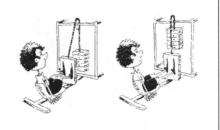

Figure 10–16

LEG EXTENSIONS: lower thighs.
Sit on machine, feet under pads,
seat against back of knees. Hold
seat below buttocks. Raise weight
until legs are parallel to floor. If
machine can restrict knee flexion,
avoid flexion greater than 90°. If
you have chondromalacia, restrict
flexion to 30° or avoid this exercise.

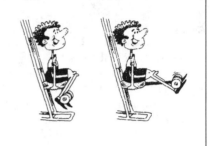

Figure 10–17

TOE RAISES: calves. Can be
done on a machine, as here,
holding dumbbells, or with a
barbell or partner on the back.
Keep back straight, legs locked,
hips in line. Raise on toes as high
as possible.

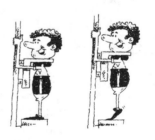

Legs/Upper Body

Figure 10–18

LEG CURLS: hamstrings. Lie
facedown, heels under top foot
pad. Hold front of machine. Curl
up as far as possible. If your
pelvis rises while curling, use a
pad or pillow under it.

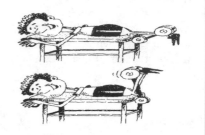

Figure 10–19

SHOULDER SHRUGS:
trapezius. Grasp a bar or
dumbbells with palms down,
hands shoulder width apart. Stand
erect. Droop shoulders as much as
possible. Raise shoulders and
rotate in a circular motion from
front to rear.

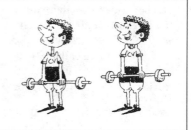

Upper Body

Figure 10–20

TRICEP CURLS: triceps. Hold
dumbbell with both hands. Raise
weight overhead to arm's length,
pushing palms upward. Keep
elbows in.

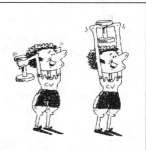

Figure 10–21

BARBELL CURLS: biceps. Hold barbell with palms up, a little more than shoulder width apart. Stand erect. Curl bar in semicircular motion. Biceps can also be worked with dumbbells.

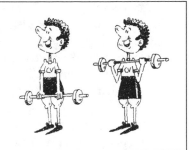

Miscellaneous

Figure 10–22

SIT-UPS: abdominals. Perform with bent knees. Straight-leg sit-ups strengthen the hip flexors, but risk back injury. Hook feet under strap of sit-up board or under piece of furniture. Don't let your shoulders go all the way down— keep tension on your abdominals. Don't flex neck.

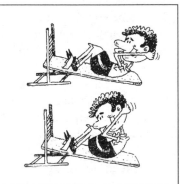

Figure 10–23

BACK EXTENSIONS: lower back. Extend body over end of high bench. End of bench at hips. Bend forward from the waist, and extend to the horizontal or just slightly farther. When you can do 20 easily, hold weight behind your head.

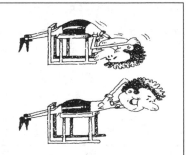

MEASURE YOUR PROGRESS

You've trained hard for a few months and wonder, has it been worthwhile? Evaluating progress and monitoring training help improvement.

GOALS HELP PROGRESS

The more specific your goals, and the more you break down those goals into components, into steps, the easier it may be to achieve those goals.

Goals can be vague, and semi-serious. You might say you want to ride to relieve stress and make more friends. After a few months, you may say, "Well I still have the same old stress on the job, but I am feeling a little more relaxed and I have nine friends now where I only had two friends before!" So you've improved!

Your goals may be more defined. You may want to ride the "B" club ride, and not get dropped. You may want to beat some guy up the local climb at the end of the ride. If you do it, it is easy to acknowledge that you've met your goal.

Getting there can be broken down into different parts: the endurance to last the length of the ride, the aerobic effort needed to stay in contention on the climb, and the anaerobic effort to sprint the last 100 meters to crest the top ahead of Joe Cool.

The more you can break down your goals into specific steps, the easier it may be to assess your progress and achieve your goals. I have seen the technique of riding a 1-kilometer track race broken down into 73 steps!

Let's take an example of a specific goal: an athlete whose goal is medaling in the time trial at the Masters Nationals.

How can we break down that endpoint? Time trialing requires certain physical ability, equipment, and mental ability. These factors can in turn be subdivided. Aerobic capacity and leg strength are the chief physical abilities. Aerobic capacity and leg strength can be measured, but most of us don't have the equipment to measure this directly. Training for aerobic and anaerobic power are discussed earlier in this chapter. Equipment needs and mental ability are discussed in Part Four.

RECORDS SHOW PROGRESS

We can get some idea from monitoring our progress during mock time trials. Here are some figures from the stationary trainer:

Table 10–4

Date	Time	Gear	Cadence	Distance	Mile/Minute
2/25	16 min	52/15	80	5.98	0.374
3/3	18 min	52/15	84	7.17	0.398
3/7	25 min	52/15	85	10.10	0.404
3/10	20 min	52/15	87	8.21	0.410
3/17	20 min	52/15	88	8.24	0.412

Is this athlete progressing? After 3 weeks of training, the athlete has ridden more than 10% faster. Other factors must be kept in mind. What was the workout load prior to the time trial? Was the athlete equally rested? Was training performed at the same time of day?

Apart from the March 7 session, all workouts were done at the same time of day, with the same warm-up. The athlete decreased his mileage from 300 to 200 miles weekly during this period of time. Some of the improvement may be related to decreasing mileage.

What other data can we analyze? Before the time trial, the athlete does a couple of isolated leg-training sessions.

Table 10–5

		Average Cadence	
Date	Gear	Left Leg	Right Leg
2/25	52/11	40 rpm	40 rpm
3/3	52/11	44 rpm	46 rpm
3/10	52/11	44 rpm	R leg injured
3/17	52/11	46 rpm	48 rpm

Here is confirming evidence of improvement. Isolated-leg training is related to leg strength. And the average rpm have increased with the same load over the 3 weeks. Leg strength is on the rise.

WHAT ABOUT RECOVERY?

Table 10–6

	Heart Rate				
	At End	Seconds after End of Effort			
Date	of Effort	30	60	90	120
2/25	no data				
3/3	177	156	140	120	107
3/10	181	159	136	116	104
3/17	183	155	134	121	108

Recovery is consistent. Heart rate falls at about the same rate after each week's effort. (This athlete was fit to begin with.)

CONCLUSION

We have good evidence that the athlete is faster, stronger, and recovering as well at the end of this month's review. The program appears to be working!

Part Three

STATIONARY TRAINING

CHAPTER 11

Trainer Basics and Sample Workouts

Why Stationary Trainers?

Stationary trainers provide the racer, the athlete, and the occasional bicycle rider many different opportunities. Some of the benefits of stationary trainers are difficult to obtain in any other way. They have some terrific advantages:

FUN

Don't let anyone tell you differently—stationary trainers are a blast. The secret is in knowing how to have fun: You must have a goal. With a workout plan in place, you can watch yourself as you improve session by session. With suitable objectives and plans, anyone can improve their performance. What's more fun than seeing your improvement?

TIME EFFICIENT

You get home from work; you have an hour to work out. If you ride your bike, it may take you 15–20 minutes to get to a road suitable for your planned workout—that hill you need to climb or that long straightaway without any traffic lights. With travel time home again, you might not get much done in that hour. With a trainer at home, you can get all the workout you need in 60 minutes.

CONVENIENT, INEXPENSIVE

For $100 you can ride at home, without the monthly fees or initiation costs of a gym, without the worry about the availability of equipment. Your bike fits you correctly; no adjustments are needed. Bad weather doesn't hinder you. You can always ride.

FITNESS

Stationary trainers work. They help to train you. They specifically train the aspects of fitness you need. Fitness improves—predictably.

HARD WORKOUT

Many of us love the feeling of our bodies working hard. Whether it is called exercise high, endorphins, whatever, working out is satisfying. Trainer workouts allow a hard workout.

With busy roads and intersections, potholes, and barking dogs, it is difficult to work to your potential, to your maximum. Trainers allow a hard, uninterrupted workout.

BICYCLING SPECIFIC

When bicycle racers can't ride they sometimes find alternative outlets for their energies. They may choose skiing or skating for cross-training in the winter. These are good choices for cyclists. Such activities are aerobic and use the legs. Still, there is no substitute for bicycle riding for a cyclist.

PRECISE WORKOUT

Top-end performance riders want to fine-tune their workouts. Runners have the track, and swimmers the lap pool, in which to time their efforts. The trainer allows the cyclist to precisely time, monitor, and tune the effort.

MOTIVATING

Trainers allow precise monitoring of performance. With suitable goals, the measured successes you achieve are extremely motivating.

As you observe your own progress and reach goals, further goals can be planned, goals that originally could only have been dreams.

SOCIAL

For most people, riding a trainer is a solitary experience. It need not be that way. I do it differently.

Trainers allow faster riders to ride with slower ones. Riders can perform an entire workout together.

Thursday nights for the last few years have been social hours chez Baker. Stationary trainer workouts are run with up to 75 riders in each session. Thursday nights, on stationary trainers, are the only nights some of these riders ride with friends!

Types of Trainers

Get a conventional trainer, where you mount your bike after taking off the front wheel, or a "track stand" type of trainer, where your rear wheel is cradled and your front wheel is left on. Conventional trainers are more stable but less portable than "track stand" trainers.

ROLLERS NOT SUITABLE

Rollers are fine for some workouts: warm-ups, spin techniques, some balance development. They are inferior for strength training, and less than optimal for aerobic training.

The trainer you use for these sessions must allow for a wide range of effort. Some exercises simulating hill climbing call for the raising of your front end. Isolated-leg training exercises are almost impossible unless your bicycle is firmly supported. For these reasons, conventional rollers are not practical.

NOT LIFECYCLES

Lifecycles are a heavy-duty type of stationary exercise bike found in gyms. We simulate hills by raising the fronts of our trainers on blocks. Lifecycles can't be used for this particular exercise. Also, Lifecycles are rarely set up to position you correctly, it's hard to effectively pull up, and ventilation is usually a problem in gyms. Simply put, Lifecycle workouts are not ideal.

FANS PREFERRED TO MAGNETIC RESISTANCE

You'll need some resistance device. Resistance devices are either fan or magnetic. Fans are cheaper, but noisier.

The magnetic type can give more resistance than the single- or double-fan setup. By varying the pressure that your rear tire exerts against the roller of the resistance device you can vary the workload considerably. The resistance of the fan setup is usually adequate for all but very strong riders in a few specific instances.

In my experience, magnetic resistance trainers perform imperfectly. The "magnet" seems lumpy. As effort and cadence increase the magnetic resistance does not vary, so you don't get the right "road feel." Mags feel easier to pedal as you work harder, rather than increasing their resistance.

Quietness—a real advantage of mags—isn't enough to offset the disadvantages. Get a fan resistance device.

NO SOFT TIRES

Avoid soft tires such as Continental tires on trainers. They are great tires for racing, but they wear out on trainers after only a couple of sessions.

Stationary Trainer Setup

USE AN OLD BIKE

You want an old bike because trainers, when you work hard, spell disaster to bicycles.

Without the bike's moving freely underneath you, enormous pressures are generated on the bicycle. The bike you use on the trainer gets wet with sweat, and rusted. The headset, with the bike always "going" straight ahead, gets grooved. Click shifting is fine for derailleurs, but you don't need click steering!

For these and many other reasons, don't use a good bike for this. Do have the bike set up identically to your regular road bike.

GEARING

Gears are found on the front—the *chain rings* attached to the right crank— and on the rear—the *cogs* found on the right side of the rear wheel. There are usually two chain rings. The chain rings commonly have from 39 to 53 teeth. There are usually 7 or 8 cogs. The cogs usually have 12 to 28 teeth. The combination of front/rear gearing is called a gear ratio, 39/28 being the easiest, 53/12 being the hardest.

Although almost any gear setup can be made to work, the type of cog setup that has worked best for most of my riders is a 12-13-14-15-16-17-20-28. If you have a 7-cog system, omit the 17 cog.

The closely spaced high gears allow one to precisely tune the hard efforts. The large 28 cog allows one to work on spin and leg speed exclusively without muscle strength or aerobic capacity (i.e., the lack thereof) limiting the drill.

FANS FOR COOLING

Preferably two large ones to help evaporate perspiration and to prevent dripping sweat.

When you ride at 25 miles per hour outside, and are working hard, the wind cools your body. When you train indoors, without that cooling wind, your core temperature rises and the body is operating in a non-race, physiologically suboptimal manner.

In addition, sweat ruins the bike and the floor or carpet it's on and increases odors. When your shorts are soaked, you chafe easily, get saddle sores, and can't ride. A sweatband and a towel are helpful but not enough. You need wind to help keep you dry. Buy a fan!

WATER BOTTLES

You can lose more than 5 pounds of water in an hour. If you're going for more than an hour, you need liquids.

Riding without fans, Ralph Myatt said he knew he was done when the 1.5-inch crack underneath his trainer was full of sweat. Ralph trained for Mexicali–San Felipe one year by riding 100 miles daily on his trainer. It took him a little over 3 hours to ride the 100 miles, and he lined up numerous water bottles beside him before starting. Replace your fluids!

ISOLATED-LEG TRAINING SUPPORT

Riding with one leg is a great way to build strength. It is a terrific way to strengthen pulling-up muscles you might otherwise neglect. You'll need a Spincoach, boxes, or other object on which to rest your non-working leg.

EARPLUGS

Trainers, when you are working hard, make a lot of noise.

If you wear headphones, as most do, you tend to crank up the volume to drown out the trainer, and can damage your ears.

I like to wear earplugs (specifically the dry foam type), and then have the headphones over the plugs. You hear the same relative level of music, the roller noise is diminished, and you protect your ears.

CADENCE AND HEART-RATE MONITORS

You need a computer with cadence to quantify your leg speed. With the same day-to-day trainer-resistance settings, a computer with cadence also serves as a power meter. A heart-rate monitor helps quantify the cardiovascular intensity of your efforts.

SAFETY

Make sure the bicycle is attached securely to the trainer, whether in the rear or by the front fork. Find level ground, and be cautious when first standing. When you are using electric fans, and you get soaked, avoid handling electrical connections. If you have small children around, be careful to avoid a setup where a child might approach you from behind and stick a hand in your rotating wheel.

If you are over 40, haven't been previously active, and are starting out on a vigorous program, consider a medical checkup before beginning. If you feel excessively weak, flushed, dizzy, or have palpitations or other problems, stop!

Stationary Trainer Workouts

YOU NEED A WORKOUT PLAN

The secret of falling in love with (or at least not hating) indoor training is to have a plan, a goal, a reason for riding indoors.

Many people find it hard to ride inside for more than about 20–30 minutes. Those bored with stationary training usually ride the same speed and in the same gear for their workouts. Challenging variation is required. Usually what they lack is a plan, a workout goal.

You can get something out of just getting on the bike and seeing how you feel—but with a workout plan you'll find the fitness rewards greater.

WARM-UP

Warm-ups are preludes to more specific training programs. They are also useful before races. They are invaluable when it's rainy, cold, or windy. Many track riders use trainers to keep warm between their events. With trainer warm-ups you can precisely control the effort you wish to exert.

Start in an easy gear, and about every minute increase your effort and cadence. At the end of 20 minutes you should be spinning about 120 rpm, working comfortably hard, but not all-out.

Many racers I have spoken with are surprised how good it feels to have warmed up for 20 minutes on the morning of a race, before their morning shower, breakfast, and travel to the race.

SPIN WORKOUT

Set the resistance of your trainer to the minimum setting. Have your tire just grazing the pressure roller. There is usually some room for adjustment on most trainers to obtain this slightest of loads. Choose an easy gear. Use a clock and cadence computer.

Start at 90 rpm. Increase your cadence by 5 rpm every minute. When you can't maintain the cadence for the full minute, cool down, and then do it once or twice again. Racers, if you can't get up to 150 rpm or so, it's a good thing you're doing this workout, because you need it!

SPRINT WORKOUT

It is a mistake to do repeated hard sprints without some pedal resistance. With little resistance, your interior knee ligaments (cruciates) have difficulty withstanding the rapidly opposing forces of direction. Without some external resistance you can easily bike into some knee troubles. You can ride with a high cadence on rollers, yes, but sudden and repeated accelerations can be a problem.

One of my favorite sprint workouts on a trainer is to do 8 to 16 sprints. Each effort lasts about 15–20 seconds, or about 40 pedal strokes. Half are seated, half are standing. Half are in the drops, half on the brake levers. (Although not the classical sprint position, you are often on the levers in races, need to sprint, and don't have the luxury of time to change to the more efficient drop sprinting position.) Half in, say, a 42/16, half in a 53/16. With all this variety in position and gear, it's hard to get bored before you get tired!

I take about a minute and a half between sprints to recover, with an extra minute or two every four sprints. Therefore, I do a sprint every 2 minutes, in sets of four. With a warm-up and a cool-down, and the sprints in between, this sprint workout can easily take an hour to perform.

HILL CLIMBING

What else! You put boards under the front of your trainer. About 4 inches of front elevation is good. For stability, I have drilled boards in which the front feet of the trainer sit.

A note of caution: If the front of your trainer rises more than 6 inches, it's easy to wheelie backwards. Another problem: Sometimes if you set up your trainer as the manufacturer suggests, with the rear wheel just barely sitting on the trainer roller surface, you may lose pedaling traction when standing. Also a problem: Pedal resistance, even in your biggest gear, may not be enough. You can lower the bottom bracket trainer support or increase the tension knob, if there is one, to allow for greater rear wheel/roller contact. It will be harder to pedal, and traction will not be lost.

You can sit or stand to simulate sitting or standing while climbing. I like standing on the bike, on the trainer, 4 inches up, and "climbing" for 15 minutes, then changing the angle by raising the front another 2 inches (for a total of 6 inches) for another 15 minutes.

Of course you can do "hill" sprints and intervals too!

EASY DAY WORKOUTS

Choose an easy gear. Usually you can go 15–20 minutes without thinking about it too much or working on any specific technique. Longer than that, and you may need some diversion.

You do not want to work hard on your easy day, and the fact that you don't have a specific hard program, technique, clock/cadence/speed, or heart rate to maintain, paradoxically, makes easy day workouts mentally difficult for many riders.

Read the paper, listen to music, get an extension cord and call your friends on the telephone.

I find my interest maintained by syncopating my pedaling rhythm. Alternate emphasis by pushing down every stroke and a half, for example, then every two and a half strokes. Then, perhaps, alternate every stroke and a half pulling up.

Remember not to work too hard. Use little pressure. "We don't work hard enough on our hard days, and we work too hard on our easy days."

CRITERIUM SPRINTS OR CRITERIUM WORKOUTS

Six to 12 all-out sprints can be plenty on a dedicated sprint day. Less intense sprints or jumps out of every corner characterize criterium racing. For example, in a fast 25-lap 4-corner crit, you may find yourself doing 100 short hard efforts just to finish.

Sprint for 10–15 seconds every 30 seconds. That's 10 seconds on, 20 seconds off, twice a minute. Do this for 20 minutes. That is 40 jumps!

You'll be amazed at your criterium and overall improvement.

STRENGTH WORKOUTS

Use the biggest gear you can maintain for at least 3 minutes. Perform 2 to 4 repeats. Unlike interval workouts, where your goal is speed, here you can let your cadence drop to push the biggest gear possible A cadence of 40–60 rpm is typical.

Concentrate on powering particular sections of the pedal stroke. For example, work on pushing 2 to 6 o'clock, then work on pulling 6 to 9, then work on pulling 9 to 1 o'clock, changing emphasis every 15–40 strokes depending on your desires.

Work on the muscles you need for the event you are targeting by duplicating the riding position you'll use. Do you want to improve your time trialing? Are you using forearm-supporting ("aero" or "tri") bars? You need them set up on your trainer bike. You need to work on the trainer "in the position."

INTERVAL WORKOUTS

Use a bigger gear than you do for the sprints, and ride as hard as you can maintain, for, say, 3 minutes. Use your speedometer. Use the gear that gets you going the fastest.

Ride so hard that you're exhausted at the end of the interval and can't go another 15 seconds at the same pace. Recover a few minutes. Go again, perhaps decreasing the time by 15 seconds each interval. Do about six intervals.

ISOLATED-LEG TRAINING

This is a workout routine that helps develop strength, technique, and speed. All three, plus more! (What more could one ask for?)

With clipless pedals, this is much easier to accomplish than it used to be. Click in only one leg. Rest the other on a Spincoach, stool, box, or water bottle holder; twist your leg around and rest it on a rear carrier, or just dangle it at the side—but use only one leg at a time!

Work especially on sections of your stroke, as described above, in the strength section. You tend to use a lower cadence when working on strength. But work on intervals, spin, and cadence with one leg too. Use one leg at a time for about 5 minutes, then alternate with the other.

At the beginning you might not be able to last 5 minutes with one leg. You'll get stronger with practice. You can then go back and forth for several repetitions.

There's so much to do! You could spend an hour on isolated-leg training alone!

COOL-DOWN

It's easy to forget about cool-downs. They are important for many reasons. They probably help recovery and lessen stiffness. Don't forget to spend at least several minutes cooling down.

OUTDOOR TRAINING

Take the trainer out-of-doors. Seriously. It's so much fun riding stationary trainers that sometimes you may forget the birds and trees are outdoors.

CHAPTER 12

The 12-Week Progressive Workout Series

The following 12 workouts were designed for the annual wintertime coached stationary trainer series of Cyclo-Vets, a San Diego–based masters bicycle racing club.

The workouts begin fairly easily, and progress to quite strenuous workouts.

Bicycle fitness has many aspects, including strength, speed, and aerobic and anaerobic ability. These workouts are mixtures of these different aspects of fitness. Each workout is designed to work on several of these areas.

The theme workouts which follow this 12-week progressive series are different. The theme workouts are designed to work on specific aspects of fitness, rather than on several aspects at once.

If you live in a cold climate where trainers are used for the majority of your winter workouts, use these 12 workouts as a framework for an expanded program. Once you get to workout 6, vary your workouts. Perhaps you'll want to stay with number 6 on Tuesday, and progress through the 12-week series on Thursdays. Perhaps you'll add a theme workout from Chapter 13 on a third day of the week.

Some of the suggestions found within the text are seasonal reminders for racers. If you are not using this as a wintertime series, a couple of the seasonal pointers may not apply.

Stationary Workout Log and Timechart Explained

Time	Gear	RPM	MPH
00:00	Warm-up		
01:00			
02:00			
03:00			
04:00			
05:00			
06:00			
07:00			
08:00			
09:00			
10:00			
11:00			
12:00			
13:00			
14:00			
15:00	42/17	70	14
16:00	Easy	75	15
17:00		80	16
18:00		85	17
19:00		90	18
20:00		95	19
21:00		100	20
22:00		105	21
23:00		110	22
24:00	Rest		
25:00		80	16
26:00		85	17
27:00		90	18
28:00		95	19
29:00		100	20
30:00		105	21
31:00		110	22
32:00		115	23
33:00		120	24
34:00	Rest		
35:00		80 85	
36:00		90 95	
37:00		100 105	
38:00		110 115	
39:00		120 125	
40:00		130 135	
41:00		140	
42:00	Rest		
43:00			
44:00			
45:00	42/15	40–60	Left leg ILT
46:00		40–60	Right leg ILT
47:00	Rest		
48:00	42/15	40–60	Left leg ILT
49:00		40–50	Right leg ILT
50:00	Rest		
51:00			
52:00	42/15	40–60	Left leg ILT
53:00		40–60	
54:00		40–60	Right leg ILT
55:00		40–60	
56:00	Cool-down		
57:00			
58:00			
59:00			

Figure 12–1

Day The day is recorded.		**Date** The date is recorded.				

Format	The number of the session is listed here. The general type of workout is listed. For example: Introduction to Spinning Isolated-Leg Training					
15 min	Warm-up	42/17				
8 min	Spin-up	42/17	to 110			
7 min	Spin-up	42/17	to 120			
7 min	Spin-up	42/17	to 140			
1 min	ILT	42/15	40+		2 reps	
2 min	ILT	42/15	40+			
4+ min	Cool-down	42/17				

Seconds	0″	30″	60″	90″	120″
120 rpm	153	136	108	82	74
140 rpm	167	140	112	87	75

Figure 12–2

OVERVIEW BOX

The overview box gives an "at-a-glance" summary of the entire workout. The first column breaks down the minutes, the second the type of exercise, the third typical gearing, the fourth nominal cadence and cadence ranges, and the fifth and last column additional information.

HEART-RATE BOX

The lower box is used to record your heart rate at the end of specific exercises within the workout, and every 30 seconds thereafter for 2 minutes.

In our example, the heart rate at the end of the 120 rpm spin-up was 153 bpm. After 30 seconds of rest it fell to 136. Heart rate fell to 74 bpm after 2 minutes. After the 140 rpm spin-up the heart rate was 167. It fell to 75 after 2 minutes.

TIMECHART

On the facing page, the Timechart gives a minute-by-minute account of the hour's workout. Nominal gear ratios, rpm, mph, and occasional instructions are given. "Nominal" means that the listed gears and rpm are for the average fit rider with a typical trainer setup.

The gearing is meant to give relative scale to the degree of difficulty. Many of the riders I have coached have been performing these sessions with me for years. They have developed excellent spin and are able to perform these workouts at higher rpm. Experienced racers, even though new to this trainer series, may spin quickly. New riders may not be able to spin as well so take the time to figure out where you fit in.

TRAINER SETUP

It is a mistake to compare your gearing directly to that of another rider. The trainer setup itself is an important factor in your choice of gears. The power necessary to push a 42/17 at 120 rpm can vary significantly from trainer to trainer.

CADENCE RECOMMENDED

A cadence computer is recommended. Sometimes equivalent mph values are given as a guide for those without cadence. Sometimes two or three cadence goals are given in the same minute row. At 35 minutes, 80 and 85 are listed. This means that 80 rpm are to be maintained for 30 seconds, and that a cadence of 85 rpm is to complete the minute.

WORD INSTRUCTIONS

Additional information, such as "Stand" or "Hill climbing," in the fourth column is meant to alert you to a change in workout technique. Rest time is allowed for you to change the trainer setup if necessary. Otherwise, "Rest" does not mean stop pedaling, it means pedal easily.

Learn to Spin and Isolated-Leg Training/Workout #1

Time	Gear	RPM	MPH
00:00	Warm–up		
01:00			
02:00			
03:00			
04:00			
05:00			
06:00			
07:00			
08:00			
09:00			
10:00			
11:00			
12:00	42/17	70	14
13:00	Easy	75	15
14:00		80	16
15:00		85	17
16:00		90	18
17:00		95	19
18:00		100	20
19:00		105	21
20:00		110	22
21:00	Rest		
22:00	42/17	80	16
23:00		85	17
24:00		90	18
25:00		95	19
26:00		100	20
27:00		105	21
28:00		110	22
29:00		115	23
30:00		120	24
31:00	Rest		
32:00	42/17	80	85
33:00		90	95
34:00		100	105
35:00		110	105
36:00		120	125
37:00		130	135
38:00		140	
39:00			
40:00			
41:00			
42:00	42/15	40–60	Left leg ILT
43:00	Rest		
44:00	42/15	40–60	Right leg ILT
45:00	Rest		
46:00	42/15	40–60	Left leg ILT
47:00	Rest		
48:00	42/15	40–60	Right leg ILT
49:00	Rest		
50:00			
51:00	42/15	40–60	Left leg ILT
52:00		40–60	
53:00	Rest		
54:00	42/15	40–60	Right leg ILT
55:00		40–60	
56:00	Cool–down		
57:00			
58:00			
59:00			

Figure 12–3

Workout #1		Day			Date		
Format	1st Coached Trainer Session						
	Introduction to Trainer Workouts						
	Intro. Spin, Intro. ILT						
15 min	Warm-up	42/17					
8 min	Spin-up	42/17	to 110				
7 min	Spin-up	42/17	to 120				
7 min	Spin-up	42/17	to 140				
1 min	ILT	42/15	40+		2 reps		
2 min	ILT	42/15	40+				
4+ min	Cool-down	42/17					
Seconds		0"	30"	60"	90"	120"	

Figure 12–4

WARM-UP

The session begins with a 12-minute adjustment period and warm-up. Spin easily and consistently.

HERE WE GO! SPIN-UP

From the 12th minute to the 20th minute, slowly increase your cadence. Start with around 70 rpm, and pedal 5 rpm faster every minute, so that by the 20th minute you are pedaling 110 rpm. If you can't do this, maybe you are in too hard a gear or the resistance of the trainer is too high.

CADENCE RPM ARE GUIDELINES

Remember, this is only a guideline. Riders with less leg speed may have to pedal more slowly. Experienced criterium riders may find these nominal values too slow. Adjust your trainer so that only the minimum amount of friction is present, and the gear is an easy one.

After a minute's rest, start again, starting at about 80 rpm, finishing at about 120 rpm.

After another minute's rest, do it one more time, but this time increase cadence 5 rpm every 30 seconds.

I've put 140 rpm on the Timechart. If you are a novice, 140 may be much too fast.

ISOLATED-LEG TRAINING

The next exercise is isolated-leg training—ILT. I've chosen 42/15 as a moderate gear. Remember, this is nominal. What you want is the gear that makes it very hard to complete a minute or two of one-legged riding at a cadence between 40 and 60.

I can't determine the exact gear for you. It depends on your trainer, its bearings, the size of your magnet, the size of your wind fans, your leg strength, and other factors too.

It will take several sessions to determine which gear is right for you. You'll get better quickly. Many riders can't push even the easiest gear with one leg for 2 minutes the first week.

COOL-DOWN

Don't forget to cool down for 5 minutes by riding easily.

Improve Your Spin and ILT/Workout #2

Time	Gear	RPM		MPH
00:00	Warm–up			
01:00				
02:00	42/17	60		12
03:00		70		14
04:00		75		15
05:00		80		16
06:00		85		17
07:00		90		18
08:00		95		19
09:00		100		20
10:00		105		21
11:00		110		22
12:00	Rest			
13:00				
14:00	42/17	85		17
15:00		90		18
16:00		95		19
17:00		100		20
18:00		105		21
19:00		110		22
20:00		115		23
21:00		120		24
22:00		125		25
23:00	Rest			
24:00				
25:00				
26:00	52/15	50–60		Left leg ILT
27:00		50–60		
28:00	Rest			
29:00		50–60		Right leg ILT
30:00		50–60		
31:00	Rest			
32:00	52/14	40–50		Left leg ILT
33:00		40–50		
34:00		40–50		
35:00	Rest			
36:00		40–50		Right leg ILT
37:00		40–50		
38:00		40–50		
39:00	Rest			
40:00				
41:00				
42:00	42/17	85		
43:00		90		
44:00		100		
45:00		100		
46:00		100		
47:00		100		
48:00		110		
49:00		110		
50:00		110		
51:00		110		
52:00		115	120	
53:00		125	130	
54:00		135	140	
55:00	HR	HR		
56:00	HR	HR	HR	
57:00				
58:00	Cool–down			
59:00				

Figure 12–5

Workout #2		Day		Date		
Format	2nd Coached Trainer Session Spin, ILT					
15 min	Warm-up	42/17	60–110			
9 min	Spin-up	42/17	85–125			
2 min	ILT	52/15	40+			
3 min	ILT	52/14	40+			
10 min	Spin	42/17	100+			
5 min	Spin-up	42/17	to 140			
4+ min	Cool-down	42/17				
Seconds		0″	30″	60″	90″	120″
140 rpm (Arnie's example)		167	140	112	87	75

Figure 12–6

NOMINAL GUIDELINES

Remember, rpm and gears are nominal. "Nominal" means something in name only. The gears you can spin and the cadence you can turn must be determined by you. The guidelines are only suggestions.

If you are not a spinner, you may have rpm 10 fewer than nominal. During spinning workouts, you'll want only the slightest amount of resistance on your trainer. You will need enough pressure on your trainer to keep traction.

A spin-up is incorporated into the warm-up.

ISOLATED LEG TRAINING

With ILT and almost all other efforts, you'll want a harder effort. Increase the pressure or setting of your friction device, or use a bigger gear. As you push with one leg, pull up with the arm on the same side.

I've nominally increased the gear to 52/15 and 52/14.

Ideally, you'll use the same increased setting from workout to workout to be able to finely tune increased efforts and gauge your performance. Chart your workout!

ILT gains are fast for most people. Improvement is easily shown after four or five sessions.

ILT DOESN'T RAISE HEART RATE

It's not necessary to check heart rate at the end of ILT sessions because ILT is a strength exercise, not an aerobic one. It doesn't raise heart rate that much.

START MONITORING HEART RATE

The last spinning exercise should raise your heart rate much more!

Start monitoring your heart rate after aerobic efforts. Take your heart rate at the end of hard aerobic efforts, and monitor it every 30 seconds for 2 minutes. This will give you some idea of your recovery and fitness. I usually pedal easily after the interval ends for a few seconds, and then stop pedaling and completely relax while watching my heart rate fall.

COOL-DOWN

Don't forget to cool down. Let yourself gradually and slowly decrease your cadence. Pedal with hardly any pressure on the cranks. End the session breathing normally.

Get Off Your Rear End, Hills Are Here/Workout #3

Time	Gear	RPM		MPH
00:00	42/17	60		12
01:00		70		14
02:00		75		15
03:00		80		16
04:00		85		17
05:00		90		18
06:00		95		19
07:00		100		20
08:00		105		21
09:00		110		22
10:00		115		23
11:00		120		24
12:00	Rest			
13:00				
14:00				
15:00	52/15	50–60		Left leg ILT
16:00		50–60		
17:00				
18:00		50–60		Right leg ILT
19:00		50–60		
20:00				
21:00	Rest			
22:00	52/14	40–50		Left leg ILT
23:00		40–50		
24:00		40–50		
25:00				
26:00		40–50		Right leg ILT
27:00		40–50		
28:00		40–50		
29:00				
30:00	Rest			
31:00				
32:00	52/15	50		Stand, raise 4 in.
33:00		50		
34:00		50		
35:00		50		
36:00		50		
37:00		50		Sit, if needed.
38:00		50		
39:00		50		
40:00		50		
41:00				
42:00				
43:00	42/17	90	95	Sit.
44:00		100	105	
45:00		110		
46:00		110		
47:00		110		
48:00		110		
49:00		110		
50:00		110		
51:00		110		
52:00		110		
53:00		110		
54:00		100	110	
55:00		115	120	
56:00		125	130	
57:00		135	140	
58:00	HR	HR		
59:00	HR	HR	HR	

Figure 12–7

Workout #3	Day		Date		
Format	3rd Coached Trainer Session				
	Spin, ILT				
	Intro. Hills				
15 min	Warm-up	42/17	60–120		
3 min	ILT	52/15	50+		
4 min	ILT	52/14	40+		
5–10 min	Stand	52/15	50		
10 min	Spin	42/17	110		
5 min	Spin-up	42/17	to 140		

	0″	30″	60″	90″	120″
Seconds					
140 rpm (Arnie's example)	167	140	106	87	89

Figure 12–8

ESTABLISH YOUR SETTINGS AND GEARS

During spinning workouts, you'll want only the slightest amount of resistance on your trainer. You will need enough pressure on your trainer to keep traction. With ILT and hill simulation, you'll want a harder effort. Increase the pressure or setting of your friction device. Ideally, you'll use the same increased setting from workout to workout. This will allow you to finely tune increased efforts and gauge your performance.

TRAIN SPECIFICALLY

If you want to work on climbing, do ILT sitting upright. If you wish to work on time trialing, do ILT in your aerobars or the drops. If you are not sure, try one set one way, one set the other way. When you switch from your left leg to your right, use both legs for about 10 seconds in between to avoid cramping.

RAISE THE FRONT OF YOUR TRAINER FOR HILL WORK

Climbing simulation is done with a 4×4 (about 20 inches long) under the front of your trainer, or under your front wheel. Be sure your bicycle is firmly attached to your trainer. Stand up. If you can't stand for the entire 10 minutes, that's okay. Build up to it in future sessions. When you must, sit down. Keep going. If you feel recovered, and the 10-minute exercise is not yet over, stand again. Experiment with your gearing so that you must work hard to achieve 50 rpm.

SPIN, HOLD IT, THEN SPIN-UP

With the last spin workout, start pedaling at about 100 rpm. If after a few minutes you feel you will be able to maintain a faster cadence, increase it by 5 rpm every couple of minutes to a maximum of 120 rpm. Hold and maintain your cadence. A minute before the spin-out begins, back off to 100 rpm. Increase your spin as able up to 140 rpm. If you can't spin that fast, keep spinning as fast as you can until the exercise is completed. If you can spin faster, start at a faster rate next week.

START HEART-RATE MONITORING

Notice your heart rate at the end of the spin-up exercise. Note your recovery every 30 seconds for 2 minutes. As fitness increases, your heart rate will recover more quickly with the same level of exertion. In order for the readings to be meaningful, rest in the same way after exercises in which you monitor your heart-rate recovery. Sitting up and pedaling slowly may result in heart rates 20 beats higher than rates noted while resting in the aerobars and not pedaling.

COOL-DOWN

Don't forget to spin slowly and cool down after the workout.

Last Week Too Easy? Start Intervals/Workout #4

Time	Gear	RPM	MPH
00:00	42/17	60	12
01:00		70	14
02:00		75	15
03:00		80	16
04:00		85	17
05:00		90	18
06:00		95	19
07:00		100	20
08:00		105	21
09:00		110	22
10:00		115	23
11:00		120	24
12:00	Rest		
13:00			
14:00			
15:00	52/15	50–60	Left leg ILT
16:00		50–60	
17:00		50–60	
18:00		50–60	Right leg ILT
19:00		50–60	
20:00		50–60	
21:00	Rest		
22:00	52/14	40–50	Left leg ILT
23:00		40–50	
24:00		40–50	
25:00		40–50	
26:00		40–50	Right leg ILT
27:00		40–50	
28:00		40–50	
29:00		40–50	
30:00	Rest		
31:00			
32:00	52/15	50	Stand, raise 4 in.
33:00		50	
34:00		50	
35:00		50	
36:00		50	
37:00		70	First 15 sec only.
38:00		70	" "
39:00		70	" "
40:00		70	" "
41:00		70	Last 30 sec. Sit.
42:00	HR	HR	
43:00	HR	HR	HR
44:00			
45:00	42/17	90	
46:00		100	
47:00			
48:00			
49:00			
50:00		110	
51:00			
52:00			
53:00			
54:00		100	110
55:00		115	120
56:00		125	130
57:00		135	140
58:00	HR	HR	
59:00	HR	HR	HR

Figure 12–9

Workout #4		Day		Date		
Format	4th Coached Trainer Session Spin, ILT, Hills Intro. Intervals					
15 min	Warm-up	42/17	60–120			
3 min	ILT	52/15	50+			
4 min	ILT	52/14	40+			
5 min	Stand	52/15	50			
5 min	Stand	52/15	70+		15" q60"*	
10 min	Spin	42/17	110			
5 min	Spin-up	42/17	to 140		5rpm q30"	
Seconds		0"	30"	60"	90"	120"
Last 30" interval						
140 rpm						

*q = every—in this case, stands for 15 seconds every minute and Spin-up 5 rpm every 30 seconds.
Figure 12–10

THINK ABOUT GOALS

Take some time and set your personal goals for the season. Work on losing weight now if you are overweight!

Our warm-up is now established. We increase cadence 5 rpm every minute till we're spinning 120 rpm.

START PACING ILT

You should now have an excellent idea what gear you should be pushing for ILT. Notice your cadence throughout your ILT interval. Determine your average cadence for the interval. Read the material on pacing which appears in Chapter 19.

CLIMBING

With a block of wood under the front of your trainer, stand up. If you were able to stand the entire 10 minutes last time, try to perform five intervals. If you couldn't stand 10 minutes last session, stand as long as you can, and don't worry about the intervals.

CLIMBING INTERVALS

Start intervals gently, by increasing standing hill climbing cadence 20 rpm for 15 seconds every minute starting at the beginning of the 6th, 7th, 8th, and 9th minutes of our 10-minute hill exercise.

Increase cadence for a total of 30 seconds at the end of the 10th minute (minute 41 on the Timechart). This gives an extra 30 seconds of partial recovery before the last and longest hill effort. Don't be disappointed if you can't perform all five intervals.

WATCH HEART RATE

Monitor your heart rate as you perform the hill exercise. You will gain a better understanding of your capabilities and physiology.

Watch your heart rate at the end of hard efforts and for 2 minutes as you recover at the end of hard exercises. Record your numbers in the table. As your fitness improves, you will see your recovery improve.

SPINNING TRENDS

Spinning is the last part of the workout. If you have been regularly performing these workouts, spinning should be easier. You may have noticed this in the warm-up.

The hill climbing interval exercise is taxing. Even though your spinning may be improving, the last exercise may be quite difficult due to exhaustion from the hill intervals.

The 12-Week Progressive Workout Series

Find Your Maximum Heart Rate/Workout #5

Time	Gear	RPM	MPH
00:00	42/17	60	12
01:00		70	14
02:00		75	15
03:00		80	16
04:00		85	17
05:00		90	18
06:00		95	19
07:00		100	20
08:00		105	21
09:00		110	22
10:00		115	23
11:00		120	24
12:00	Rest		
13:00			
14:00			
15:00	52/15	50–60	Left leg ILT
16:00		50–60	
17:00		50–60	
18:00		50–60	Right leg ILT
19:00		50–60	
20:00		50–60	
21:00	Rest		
22:00	52/14	40–50	Left leg ILT
23:00		40–50	
24:00		40–50	
25:00		40–50	
26:00		40–50	Right leg ILT
27:00		40–50	
28:00		40–50	
29:00		40–50	
30:00	Rest		
31:00			
32:00	52/15	55	Stand, raise 4 in.
33:00		55	
34:00		80	20 strokes or 15 sec. Try to
35:00		80	count your strokes. Set goals
36:00		80	for the interval.
37:00		80	
38:00		80	First 15 sec only.
39:00		80	″ ″
40:00		80	″ ″
41:00		80	Last 30 sec. Sit.
42:00	HR	HR	
43:00	HR	HR	
44:00	HR		
45:00	42/17	80	
46:00		90	
47:00		100	
48:00			
49:00			
50:00		110	
51:00			
52:00			
53:00			
54:00		100	110
55:00		115	120
56:00		125	130
57:00		135	140
58:00	HR	HR	
59:00	HR	HR	HR

Figure 12–11

Workout #5	Day			Date			
Format	5th Coached Trainer Session						
	Spin, ILT, Hills, Intervals						
15 min	Warm-up	42/17	60–120				
3 min	ILT	52/15	50+				
4 min	ILT	52/14	40+				
2 min	Stand	52/15	55				
8 min	Stand	52/15	80+	15" q60"			
10 min	Spin	42/17	110				
5 min	Spin-up	42/17	to 140	5rpm q30"			
Seconds		0"	30"	60"	90"	120"	
Last 30" interval							
140 rpm							

Figure 12–12

IMPROVE LAST WEEK'S WORKOUT
The workout is the same as last week's, except that the hill climbing exercise is harder.

HARDER HILL INTERVALS
We continue intervals by increasing hill cadence 25 rpm for 15 seconds every minute for the 3rd through 9th minutes of our hill workout. The last minute of the hill workout, a double-length absolutely hardest effort of 30 seconds finishes it.

HEART-RATE GOALS
You will probably want to perform the first 5 minutes of steady standing at about 75% of your maximum heart rate. Each 15-second interval will increase your heart rate a few percentage points so that at the end of the fourth effort you will be at about 90% of your maximum heart rate.

Take your heart rate after the final 30-second interval and every 30 seconds for 2 minutes thereafter. Your last and final 30-second effort should end with your heart rate between 90% and 100% of your maximum.

If your recovery heart rate falls to under 100 bpm, or half your maximum, you are fit!

COMPARE YOUR EFFORTS TO RECORDS IN THIS BOOK
The two graphs following this fifth workout are titled Standing Intervals and Spin and Spin-up. They show heart rate vs. cadence of a fit athlete while performing the standing interval and final spin section of workout 5. Using your heart monitor, compare your readings to his to measure how fit you are. If you don't have a heart-rate monitor, consider buying or borrowing one. As you can see, it can help provide you with important information about your training and fitness.

READ AHEAD
Read the workout of the upcoming session before the workout so that you have a better idea what the workout will be. Knowing about the workout ahead of time will help you visualize it in advance, and help you concentrate on your efforts.

VISUALIZE
Be sure to read Chapter 24, Visualization. Try to incorporate some of those concepts into your efforts on the stationary trainer.

Workout #5/Heart-Rate Graph: Standing Intervals

This is a heart-rate recording of a fit athlete from the 5th workout of the 12-Week Trainer Series. Recording begins 1 minute into the drill. Recovery heart rate is monitored for 2 minutes.

THE DRILL

Elevate the front of the trainer. Push as hard a gear as possible to be able to complete the drill. Stand for 10 minutes. From the beginning of the 3rd minute, increase rpm to 80 for 15 seconds each minute.

Partially recover for 45 seconds each minute, letting cadence drop to 55 rpm. The last interval has an extra 30-second partial recovery, and lasts twice as long—30 seconds. Monitor recovery heart rate for 2 minutes.

Figure 12–13 Session 5 stationary trainer workout: standing intervals.

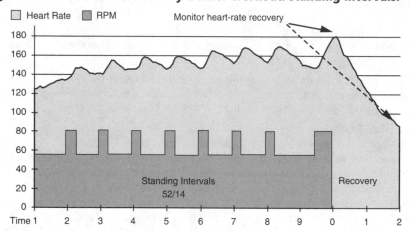

Notice:

- Heart rate lags effort by about 15 seconds.
- The heart rate rises with each 15-second interval, and falls in between.
- Each effort results in an ever-increasing heart rate during the effort and subsequent recovery period. Before the last effort, there is an extra 30 seconds of partial recovery during which heart rate drops even lower and then rises to a high of 180 after the final, long 30-second interval.
- The drill maximum heart rate achieved was 180. The physiologic maximum heart rate for *this rider* is about 190. Remember, your numbers may not be identical since everyone's max heart rate is different. Knowing your max heart rate will help you determine whether you are working hard enough.
- The extra 30 seconds of partial recovery at 9 minutes into the drill allows the athlete to begin the last interval at 147 beats per minute rather than at 154 bpm.
- Recovery is excellent, falling to 88 beats per minute in 2 minutes, or less than one-half of the drill maximum.

BONUS: RACE CORRELATION

Partial relative recovery, or the rapid descent of heart rate after an intense interval, is essential for competitive riders. Recovery times will improve as your fitness improves, which will allow you to reattack faster and more often. You'll be able to dictate the race and respond to repeated attacks.

Workout #5/Heart-Rate Graph: Spin and Spin-up

This is a heart-rate recording of a fit athlete from the 5th workout of the 12-Week Trainer Series. Recording begins 1 minute into the drill. Recovery is monitored for 2 minutes. This fit athlete had a cadence higher than our average rider from workout 5.

THE DRILL

The chart below shows the heart rate changing with cadence. The athlete pedaled at 115 rpm for 1 minute, and then held 120 rpm for 4 minutes. Cadence then dropped to 100 rpm for 30 seconds. The athlete raised cadence again by 5 rpm every 30 seconds until he held 140 rpm for 30 seconds. Heart rate was recorded during the exercise. Recovery heart rate was monitored for 2 minutes.

Figure 12–14 **Session 5 stationary trainer workout: spin and spin-up.**

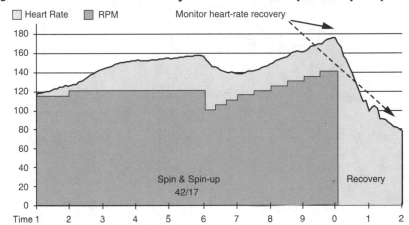

Notice:

- A gradual climb in heart rate while spinning at 120 rpm. Though the effort is constant at 120 rpm from the 2nd to the 6th minute, the heart rate "catches up" and rises gradually. There may also be a heat effect.
- The drill maximum heart rate achieved was 177. The physiologic maximum heart rate for this rider is about 190.
- The heart rate at the end of the 5th minute, after 4 minutes at 120 rpm, was 159. The heart rate at the end of the 7th minute, after spinning 120 rpm for 30 seconds, was 149. With partial recovery, spinning at 125 rpm began at a heart rate 10 beats lower than would have been the case had a minute of partial recovery not been scheduled.
- If we hadn't allowed for recovery after the 120-rpm spin section, 140 rpm could only have been achieved by an athlete with a higher maximum heart rate. If the drill heart rate reached the physiologic maximum heart rate of the athlete—before the completion of 30 seconds at 140 rpm—the athlete in this instance, with a max heart rate of 190 bpm, would probably have been too exhausted to finish the exercise.
- Recovery is excellent, falling to 78 bpm in 2 minutes, or less than one-half of the drill maximum.

Raise Your Working Heart Rate/Workout #6

Time	Gear	RPM	MPH	
00:00	42/17	60	12	
01:00		70	14	
02:00		75	15	
03:00		80	16	
04:00		85	17	
05:00		90	18	
06:00		95	19	
07:00		100	20	
08:00		105	21	
09:00		110	22	
10:00		115	23	
11:00		120	24	
12:00	Rest			
13:00				
14:00				
15:00	52/14	50		Left leg ILT
16:00		50		
17:00		50		
18:00		50		
19:00		50		Right leg ILT
20:00		50		
21:00		50		
22:00		50		
23:00	Rest			
24:00				
25:00	52/15	55		Stand, raise 4 in.
26:00		55		
27:00		80		20 strokes or 15 sec. Try to
28:00		80		count your strokes. Set goals
29:00		80		for the interval.
30:00		80		
31:00		80		First 15 sec only.
32:00		80		" "
33:00		80		" "
34:00		80		Last 30 sec. Sit.
35:00	HR	HR		
36:00	HR	HR		
37:00	HR			
38:00	52/16	85		Should be a hard-gear effort.
39:00		85		4-min time trial.
40:00		85		
41:00		85		
42:00	HR	HR		
43:00	HR	HR		
44:00	HR			
45:00	42/17	70	75	
46:00		80	90	
47:00		100		
48:00		100		
49:00		100		
50:00		110		
51:00		110		
52:00		110		
53:00		110		
54:00		100	110	
55:00		115	120	
56:00		125	130	
57:00		135	140	
58:00	HR	HR		
59:00	HR	HR	HR	

Figure 12–15

Workout #6		Day		Date		
Format	6th Coached Trainer Session					
	Spin, ILT, Hills, Intervals					
15 min	Warm-up	42/17	60–120			
4 min	ILT	52/14	50			
2 min	Stand	52/15	55+			
8 min	Stand	52/15	80+	15″ q60″		
4 min	Sit	52/16	80–90			
7 min	Spin	42/17	110			
3 min	Spin-up	42/17	to 140	5rpm q30″		
Seconds		0″	30″	60″	90″	120″
Last 30″ interval						
End of 4′ TT						
140 rpm						

Figure 12–16

WARM-UP

Warm up as before. There will be only one ILT repetition today to make room for the longer time-trial-type interval.

WORK ON HILLS

As before, a double effort of 30 seconds finishes the last minute of the hill workout. Take your heart rate at this point (the beginning of the 35th minute) and every 30 seconds for 2 minutes thereafter. Heart-rate goal at the end of the hill session is 90–95% of your maximum.

BEGIN TIME-TRIAL TRAINING

We start time-trial training today with a 4-minute effort. Choose the hardest gear you can pedal at about 85 rpm to just complete the interval. Read Chapter 19 on time trials.

BREATHING

This is our first 4-minute time trial/interval. Concentrate on your breathing pattern: I find a rhythm with one breath every one and a half strokes works well.

ASSESS YOUR PROGRESS

We're halfway through the Trainer Series. It's time to consider your strengths and weaknesses and your racing goals for the upcoming year. It's time to think about or plan for some important special events.

CONSIDER A TIME-TRIAL RACE

If you've never raced, target one of the local time trials, and plan to enter. A week or two before, simulate race day with a practice race that mimics the coming event.

TARGET YOUR SEASON GOALS

If you've raced before, target some special races in the coming season. Think about what you'll need—equipment, training, logistics. Start planning.

Experienced racers: Do you know where Nationals and Districts are? Have you called the local chamber of commerce for maps, hotel lists, etc.? Do you have a preliminary idea of the racecourses and lengths so that you can train specifically later in the spring? Schedule yourself a few hours this weekend to sit down, make lists, find motels within spitting distance of the starting line, and get organized!

Get That Heart Rate Up/Workout #7

Time	Gear	RPM		MPH
00:00	42/17	60		12
01:00		70		14
02:00		75		15
03:00		80		16
04:00		85		17
05:00		90		18
06:00		95		19
07:00		100		20
08:00		105		21
09:00		110		22
10:00		115		23
11:00		120		24
12:00	Rest			
13:00				
14:00				
15:00	52/14	50		Left leg ILT
16:00		50		
17:00		50		
18:00		50		
19:00		50		Right leg ILT
20:00		50		
21:00		50		
22:00		50		
23:00	Rest			
24:00				
25:00	52/15	55		Stand, raise 4 in.
26:00		55		
27:00		80		20 strokes or 15 sec. Try to
28:00		80		count your strokes. Set goals
29:00		80		for the interval.
30:00		80		
31:00		80		First 15 sec only.
32:00		80		" "
33:00		80		" "
34:00		80		Last 30 sec. Sit.
35:00	HR	HR		
36:00	HR	HR		
37:00	HR			
38:00	52/16	85		Should be a hard-gear effort.
39:00	52/16	85		4-min time trial.
40:00		85		
41:00		85		
42:00	HR	HR		
43:00	HR	HR		
44:00	HR			
45:00	42/17	70	75	
46:00		80	90	
47:00		100		
48:00		100		
49:00		100		
50:00		110		
51:00		110		
52:00		110		
53:00		110		
54:00		100	110	
55:00		115	120	
56:00		125	130	
57:00		135	140	
58:00	HR	HR		
59:00	HR	HR	HR	

Figure 12–17

Workout #7		Day		Date	

| Format | 7th Coached Trainer Session | | | | |
| | Spin, ILT, Hills, Intervals | | | | |

15 min	Warm-up	42/17	60–120		
4 min	ILT	52/14	50		
2 min	Stand	52/15	55+		
8 min	Stand	52/15	80+	15" q60"	
4 min	Sit	52/16	80–90		
7 min	Spin	42/17	110		
3 min	Spin-up	42/17	to 140	5rpm q30"	

Seconds	0"	30"	60"	90"	120"
Last 30" interval					
End of 4' TT					
140 rpm					

Figure 12–18

DON'T BE AFRAID TO WORK HARD
At least once a week, work absolutely as hard as you can.

- Expose yourself.
- Be vulnerable.
- Interval day is the day to do it!

A double effort of 30 seconds finishes the last minute of the hill workout. Take your heart rate at this point (35:00) and every 30 seconds for 2 minutes thereafter. Your heart-rate goal at the end of the hill session is 95% or more of your maximum.

READ MORE ON TIME TRIALING
Finish reading Chapter 19 if you didn't manage to do so last week.

This is a repeat of the last session to "dial in" your 4-minute interval effort. Read the material on intervals in Chapter 10.

Keep That Heart Rate Up/Workout #8

Time	Gear	RPM	MPH
00:00	Easy	60	12
01:00		70	14
02:00		75	15
03:00		80	16
04:00		85	17
05:00		90	18
06:00		95	19
07:00		100	20
08:00		105	21
09:00		110	22
10:00		115	23
11:00		120	24
12:00	Rest		
13:00			
14:00			
15:00	52/15	55	Stand, raise 4 in.
16:00		55	
17:00		80	20 strokes or 15 sec. Count
18:00		80	your strokes and set goals.
19:00		80	
20:00		80	
21:00		80	
22:00		80	
23:00		80	
24:00		80	Last 30 sec. Sit.
25:00	HR	HR	
26:00	HR	HR	
27:00	HR		
28:00	Rest		
29:00			
30:00	52/16	85	Should be a hard-gear effort.
31:00		85	4-min TT.
32:00		85	
33:00		85	
34:00	Rest		
35:00			
36:00	52/16	85	Should be a hard-gear effort.
37:00		85	4-min TT.
38:00		85	
39:00		85	
40:00	Rest		
41:00			
42:00	52/15	85	Should be a hard-gear effort.
43:00		85	3-min TT.
44:00		85	
45:00	HR	HR	
46:00	HR	HR	
47:00	HR		
48:00	42/17	80	
49:00		95	
50:00		110	
51:00		125	
52:00		125	
53:00		125	
54:00		100	110
55:00		115	120
56:00		125	130
57:00		135	140+
58:00	HR	HR	
59:00	HR	HR	HR

Figure 12–19

Workout #8	Day		Date	

Format — 8th Coached Trainer Session
Spin, Hills, Intervals

15 min	Warm-up	42/17	60–120	
2 min	Stand	52/15	55+	
8 min	Stand	52/15	80+	15" q60"
4 min	Sit	52/16	80–90	
4 min	Sit	52/16	80–90	
3 min	Sit	52/15	80–90	
7 min	Spin	42/17	to 125	
3 min	Spin-up	42/17	to 140	5rpm q30"

Seconds	0"	30"	60"	90"	120"
Last 30" interval					
End of 3' TT					
140 rpm					

Figure 12–20

TWO WEEKLY TRAINER WORKOUTS?

Vary your workouts. This is workout 8. If you are stationary training twice a week, don't do two number 8's. Go back and do a number 5 (ILT and standing) for one of your sessions.

HEART-RATE GOALS

In the last minute of the hill section a double effort of 30 seconds finishes the effort (24:00). Take your heart rate at this point and every 30 seconds for 2 minutes thereafter. Heart-rate goal at the end of the hill session is 92% or more of your maximum. Same thing at the end of the spin-up at 58:00.

INTERVALS

Intervals of 3 to 4 minutes are to be done in the hardest gear you can push to complete the interval and maintain a cadence of 70–95 depending upon your trainer, settings, preferences, and proclivities! If you are able to finish the 4-minute intervals without any problem, consider shifting to a harder gear for the last 3-minute effort. Record your heart rate at the end of the last time-trial interval.

READ ACCOMPANYING HEART-RATE GRAPHS

Just as in session 5, I have provided, in the next two figures, sample heart-rate graphs from a fit athlete whose max heart rate is 190. The first graph charts almost an entire session 8, while the second graph zeroes in on a time-trial section performed 1 month later. Notice the improvements in recovery and slightly higher cadence at the end of the final 3-minute time trial.

AEROBIC VS. ANAEROBIC TRAINING

Aerobic efforts are ones you can sustain. Your body uses oxygen as a component of the fuel that powers your body.

Anaerobic efforts cannot be sustained for long periods of time. The body uses up energy sources too quickly, more quickly than they are replaced, and toxic chemicals, such as lactic acid, are formed.

It is a little like your bank account—if you have a good cash flow, and keep on putting money regularly into your account, you can make steady withdrawals. That's aerobic metabolism. Take out huge clumps of money without putting cash back into your account, and pretty soon you're overdrawn, in debt, and in trouble! That's anaerobic metabolism.

Be sure you've read the material on aerobic training and anaerobic training that appears in Chapter 10.

Workout #8/Heart-Rate Graph: Keep That Heart Rate Up

As I mentioned, this is a heart-rate and cadence recording of a fit athlete from the Cyclo-Vets Thursday evening coached Trainer Series. Recording begins 15 minutes into the workout.

THE DRILL

A 15-minute warm-up preceded this recording. From the 15th minute to the 25th minute of the session, engage in 10 minutes of standing on the trainer. Push a hard gear at 55 rpm, with the front of the trainer elevated. At the beginning of the 3rd minute, increase rpm to 80 for 15 seconds. Partially recover for 45 seconds. The last interval has an extra 30 seconds of partial recovery, and lasts 30 seconds.

Then 5 minutes of recovery; two 4-minute time trials in as hard a gear as you can push at 85 rpm starting at the 30th minute of the session, with 2-minute recovery after each; and a 3-minute time trial at the same or slightly higher rpm.

Recover for about 5 minutes, gradually spinning up to 120 rpm. Hold 120 rpm for 4 minutes and then, from 100 rpm, do a spin-up to 140 rpm increasing cadence by 5 rpm every 30 seconds.

All riders are encouraged to monitor their heart rates and 2-minute recovery at the end of selected work efforts.

Figure 12–21 **Session 8 stationary trainer workout: sprints, intervals, spin.**

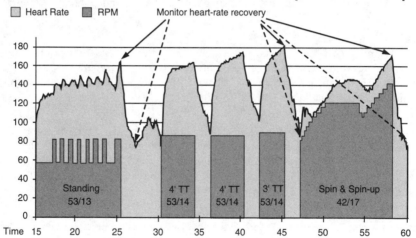

Notice:

- During the standing (climbing) drill, the heart rate rises with each 15-second interval, and falls in between. Each effort results in a trend to ever-increasing heart rate and the fall is to a level higher than before.
- Heart rates achieved in this drill were suboptimal for aerobic/anaerobic training. The athlete found his 13-tooth cog too easy, and his 11 too hard. His effort was insufficient.
- Efforts during 3- and 4-minute time trials were better.
- The physiologic maximum heart rate for this rider is about 190. The session maximum heart rate achieved was 182, or about 96% of max. During the 3- and 4-minute time trials, heart rate rises rapidly to over 160 bpm, or about 85% of max.
- Recovery is excellent.

Workout #12/Heart-Rate Graph: Time-Trial Intervals

This is a heart-rate and cadence recording from session 12 performed by the same athlete, who had now been interval training for more than a month. Contrast this recording with the same time-trial interval section during workout 8 on the facing page.

THE DRILL

A warm-up and sprint workout preceded this recording. Two 4-minute time trials in as hard a gear one can push at 85 rpm starting at the 30th minute of the session, with 2-minute recovery after each. Three-minute time trial at the same or slightly higher rpm.

Recovery and a spin workout followed this drill. All riders are encouraged to monitor their heart rates and 2-minute recovery at the end of selected work efforts.

Figure 12–22 **Session 12 stationary trainer workout: time-trial intervals.**

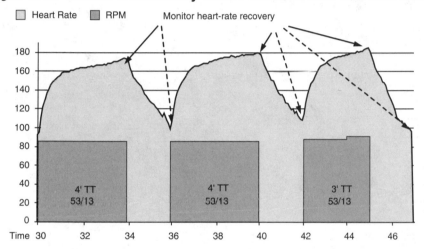

Notice:

- Efforts during 3- and 4-minute time trials train aerobic and anaerobic systems. The athlete pedaled at a cadence of 85 rpm for the two 4-minute intervals. He rode 88 rpm for the first 2 minutes of the 3-minute interval and then nudged up to 90 rpm for the final minute.
- The time trials in this session are accomplished in a bigger gear and with higher heart-rate levels than are those in session 8.
- The physiologic max heart rate for this rider is about 190. The session max heart rate was 184, about 97% of physiological max.
- During the 3- and 4-minute time trials, heart rate rises rapidly to over 157 bpm, or about 83% of max.
- Fit athletes can time-trial at 92% of maximum heart rate under optimal rest, fitness, and race conditions for 45 to 60 minutes. This athlete's 92% level is reached at a heart rate of 174. The first effort barely reached this level. One-half of the remaining interval time was spent at or above this threshold. Since heart rate lags effort in anaerobic work, this represents excellent work.
- Recovery is very good, measured on three occasions, each time falling to about 100.

Dial in Your Aerobic Threshold/Workout #9

Time	Gear	RPM		MPH
00:00	Easy	60		12
01:00		70		14
02:00		75		15
03:00		80		16
04:00		85		17
05:00		90		18
06:00		95		19
07:00		100		20
08:00		105		21
09:00		110		22
10:00		115		23
11:00		120		24
12:00	Rest			
13:00				
14:00				
15:00	52/15	55		Stand, raise 4 in.
16:00		55		
17:00		80		20 strokes or 15 sec. Count
18:00		80		your strokes and set goals.
19:00		80		
20:00		80		
21:00		80		
22:00		80		
23:00		80		
24:00		80		Last 30 sec. Sit.
25:00	HR	HR		
26:00	HR	HR	HR	
27:00	Rest			
28:00				
29:00				
30:00	52/16	85		Should be a hard-gear effort.
31:00		85		4-min TT.
32:00		85		
33:00		85		
34:00	Rest			
35:00				
36:00	52/16	85		Should be a hard-gear effort.
37:00		85		4-min TT.
38:00		85		
39:00		85		
40:00	Rest			
41:00				
42:00	52/15	85		Should be a hard-gear effort.
43:00		85		3-min TT.
44:00		85		
45:00	HR	HR		
46:00	HR	HR	HR	
47:00				
48:00	42/17	80		
49:00		95		
50:00		110		
51:00		125		
52:00		125		
53:00		125		
54:00		100	110	
55:00		115	120	
56:00		125	130	
57:00		135	140+	
58:00	HR	HR		
59:00	HR	HR	HR	

Figure 12–23

Workout #9		Day		Date		
Format	9th Coached Trainer Session Spin, Hills, Intervals					
15 min	Warm-up	42/17	60–120			
2 min	Stand	52/15	55+			
8 min	Stand	52/15	80+	15" q60"		
4 min	Sit	52/16	80–90			
4 min	Sit	52/16	80–90			
3 min	Sit	52/15	80–90			
7 min	Spin	42/17	to 125			
3 min	Spin-up	42/17	to 140	5rpm q30"		
Seconds		0"	30"	60"	90"	120"
Last 30" interval						
End of 3' TT						
140 rpm						

Figure 12–24

HEART-RATE GOALS

Heart rate at the end of the hill session should reach 92% or more of your maximum. Same thing at the end of the 3-minute interval at 45:00 and spin-out at 58:00.

INTERVAL GEARING REMINDER

Intervals of 3 to 4 minutes are done in the hardest gear you can push to complete the interval and maintain a cadence of 70–95. This depends upon your trainer, settings, preferences, and proclivities.

WORK ON BREATHING

Concentrate on your breathing in the time-trial sections. Start breathing in your time trial rhythm 5 seconds before the interval starts.

HEART-RATE REGISTRATION

Review the 3- and 4-minute time-trial heart-rate registration of an athlete from session 12+ of the Trainer Series, which appears before this workout. Notice how improvement occurred for this already fit athlete over the course of a month's training.

Get a Jump/Workout #10

Time	Gear	RPM		MPH
00:00	Easy	60		12
01:00		70		14
02:00		75		15
03:00		80		16
04:00		85		17
05:00		90		18
06:00		95		19
07:00		100		20
08:00		105		21
09:00		110		22
10:00		115		23
11:00		120		24
12:00		125		25
13:00				
14:00				
15:00				
16:00	52/17	80+		
17:00		140+		35 strokes or 15 sec. Count
18:00		140+		your strokes and set goals.
19:00		140+		
20:00		140+		
21:00		140+		
22:00		140+		
23:00		140+		
24:00		140+		30 sec sprint.
25:00	HR	HR		
26:00	HR	HR	HR	
27:00				
28:00				
29:00				
30:00	52/16	85		Should be a hard-gear effort.
31:00		85		4-min TT.
32:00		85		
33:00		85		
34:00	Rest			
35:00				
36:00	52/16	85		Should be a hard-gear effort.
37:00		85		4-min TT.
38:00		85		
39:00		85		
40:00	Rest			
41:00				
42:00	52/15	85		Should be a hard-gear effort.
43:00		85		3-min TT.
44:00		85		
45:00	HR	HR		
46:00	HR	HR	HR	
47:00				
48:00	42/17	80		
49:00		95		
50:00		110		
51:00		125		
52:00		125		
53:00		125		
54:00		100	110	
55:00		115	120	
56:00		125	130	
57:00		135	140+	
58:00	HR	HR		
59:00	HR	HR	HR	

Figure 12–25

Workout #10		Day			Date	
Format	10th Coached Trainer Session					
	Spin, Hills, Intervals					
	Intro. Sprints					
15 min	Warm-up	42/17	60–125			
10 min	Jumps	52/17	140+			
4 min	Interval	52/16	80–90			
4 min	Interval	52/16	80–90			
3 min	Interval	52/15	80–90			
7 min	Spin	42/17	to 125			
3 min	Spin-up	42/17	to 140	5rpm q30″		

Seconds	0″	30″	60″	90″	120″
Last 30″ interval					
End of 3′ TT					
140 rpm					

Figure 12–26

JUMPS

Jumps are to be done in a gear that provides some resistance.

After a minute in this gear, jump hard up to speed, and hold that fast cadence for 15 seconds. It may help to count your strokes. If you can achieve 140 rpm you'll get 35 strokes in 15 seconds.

Try to maintain or increase the number of strokes you achieve with each repetition. Perform a 15-second jump every minute for seven repetitions. After the seventh jump, give yourself an extra 30 seconds of recovery.

The eighth and last jump, in the last half of the last minute of the exercise, is for 30 seconds. Aim for the fastest possible acceleration up to maximum cadence. Jump!

TIME-TRIAL INTERVALS

Intervals of 3 to 4 minutes are done in the hardest gear you can push to complete the interval and maintain a cadence of 70–95. This depends upon your trainer, settings, preferences, and proclivities. HR readings should be 90% or more of max.

WORK ON FORM

With each time-trial interval concentrate on a different aspect of your form. For example, focus on pulling up, or keeping your knees in toward the top tube, or your back flat, or your elbows in, or your upper body relaxed, or your breathing rhythm. Work on technique, you'll go faster!

Work Your Jump/Workout #11

Time	Gear	RPM	MPH
00:00	Easy	60	12
01:00		70	14
02:00		75	15
03:00		80	16
04:00		85	17
05:00		90	18
06:00		95	19
07:00		100	20
08:00		105	21
09:00		110	22
10:00		115	23
11:00		120	24
12:00		125	25
13:00			
14:00			
15:00			
16:00	52/17	80+	
17:00		140+	35 strokes or 15 sec. Count
18:00		140+	your strokes and set goals.
19:00		140+	
20:00		140+	
21:00		140+	
22:00		140+	
23:00		140+	
24:00		140+	30-sec sprint.
25:00	HR	HR	
26:00	HR	HR	HR
27:00			
28:00			
29:00			
30:00	52/16	85	Should be a hard-gear effort.
31:00		85	4-min TT.
32:00		85	
33:00		85	
34:00	Rest		
35:00			
36:00	52/16	85	Should be a hard-gear effort.
37:00		85	4-min TT.
38:00		85	
39:00		85	
40:00	Rest		
41:00			
42:00	52/15	85	Should be a hard-gear effort.
43:00		85	3-min TT.
44:00		85	
45:00	HR	HR	
46:00	HR	HR	HR
47:00			
48:00	42/17	80	
49:00		100	
50:00		125	
51:00		125	
52:00		125	
53:00		125	
54:00		100	110
55:00		115	120
56:00		125	130
57:00		135	140+
58:00	HR	HR	
59:00	HR	HR	HR

Figure 12–27

Workout #11		Day		Date		
Format	11th Coached Trainer Session					
	Spin, Sprints, Intervals					
15 min	Warm-up	42/17	60–125			
10 min	Jumps	52/17	140+			
4 min	Interval	52/16	80–90			
4 min	Interval	52/16	80–90			
3 min	Interval	52/15	80–90			
7 min	Spin	42/17	to 125			
3 min	Spin-up	42/17	to 140	5rpm q30″		

Seconds	0″	30″	60″	90″	120″
Last 30″ interval					
End of 3′ TT					
140 rpm					

Figure 12–28

JUMPS

Jumps are to be done in a gear that provides some resistance. After a minute in this gear, jump hard up to speed, and hold that fast cadence for 15 seconds. It may help to count your strokes. If you can achieve 140 rpm you'll get 35 strokes in 15 seconds.

Try to maintain or increase the number of strokes you achieve with each repetition. Perform a 15-second jump every minute for four repetitions. Then vary the duration of the last four jumps from 5 to 30 seconds. Have a friend, spouse or coach tell you when to start and when to stop. You should perform each of these as if it will be for only 5 seconds. When the effort lasts longer, you will be very tired, having anticipated a much shorter effort.

You will get much fitter!

TIME-TRIAL INTERVALS

Intervals of 3 to 4 minutes are done in the hardest gear you can push to complete the interval and maintain a cadence of 70–95. This depends upon your trainer, settings, preferences, and proclivities.

HR readings should be 90% or more of max.

READ ACCOMPANYING HEART-RATE GRAPH

As in workouts 5 and 8, I have provided a heart-rate graph that you can use as a comparison piece to your own progress.

WORK ON FORM

With each time-trial interval concentrate on a different aspect of your form. For example, focus on pulling up, or keeping your knees in toward the top tube, or your back flat, or your elbows in, or your upper body relaxed, or your breathing rhythm. Work on technique and you'll go faster!

Workout #11/Heart-Rate Graph: Work Your Jump

This is a heart-rate and partial cadence recording of a fit athlete performing workout 11. Recording begins 5 minutes into the workout.

THE DRILL

Five minutes of the 13-minute warm-up preceded the recording. From the beginning of the 16th minute to the end of the 24th minute of the session, a sprint workout. In a moderate gear, after the first minute, 15 seconds of all-out effort to a cadence of about 140 rpm for four sprints. Then three sprints of uncertain duration. In this session the sprints were 5, 18, and 7 seconds long. Then an extra 30 seconds of recovery, and a 30-second sprint.

Five minutes of recovery. Two 4-minute time trials in as hard a gear as one can push at 85 rpm starting at the 30th minute of the session. Two-minute recovery after each. Three-minute time trial at the same or slightly higher rpm.

Recovery period for about 5 minutes, gradually spinning up to 120 rpm, which is held for 4 minutes, and then, from 100 rpm a spin-up to 140 rpm, increasing cadence by 5 rpm every 30 seconds.

Figure 12–29 **Session 11 stationary trainer workout: spin, sprints, and intervals.**

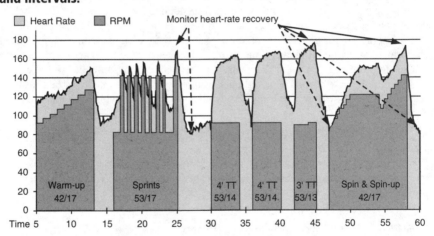

Notice:

- During the sprint drill, the heart rate rises with each 15-second interval, and falls in between. Heart rates achieved in this drill do not reach maximum levels because the effort is too short. The fifth and seventh sprints were very short, 5–7 seconds.
- Efforts during 3- and 4-minute time trials train aerobic and anaerobic systems. The athlete pedaled at a cadence of 90 rpm for the first two, then shifted to a harder gear. Time trials in this session are accomplished at the same heart-rate levels as in session 8, but cadence is up 5 rpm. The athlete is fitter.
- The physiological max heart rate for this rider is about 190. The session maximum heart rate was 176, or about 93% of max.
- During the 3- and 4-minute time trials, heart rate rises rapidly to over 160 bpm, or about 85% of max.
- Recovery is excellent.

Workout #12/Heart-Rate Graph: Master Your Jump

This is a heart-rate and partial cadence recording from a fit athlete performing workout 12.

THE WORKOUT

A 15-minute warm-up preceded this recording. From the beginning of the 15th minute to the end of the 23rd minute, a sprint workout. In a moderate gear, after the first minute, 15 seconds of all-out effort to a cadence of about 140 rpm for four sprints. Then three sprints of 20, 10, and 5 seconds. Then an extra 30 seconds of recovery, and a 30-second sprint.

Three minutes of recovery. Two 4-minute time trials in as hard a gear as one can push at 85 rpm starting at the 30th minute of the session. Two-minute recovery after each. Three-minute time trial at the same or slightly higher rpm.

Recovery for about 5 minutes, gradually spinning up to 120 rpm, which is held for 4 minutes, and then, from 100 rpm, a spin-up to 140 rpm, increasing cadence by 5 rpm every 30 seconds.

All riders are encouraged to monitor their heart rates and 2-minute recovery at the end of selected work efforts.

Figure 12–30 **Session 12 stationary trainer workout: spin, sprints, and intervals**

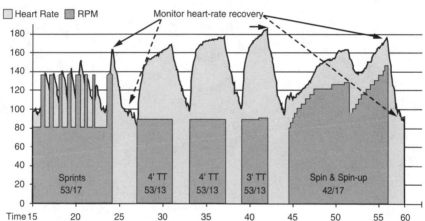

Notice:

- Heart rates achieved in the sprint drill do not reach maximum levels because the effort is too short.
- Efforts during 3- and 4-minute time trials train aerobic and anaerobic systems. The athlete pedaled at a cadence of 88 rpm. He nudged up to 90 rpm for the last minute of the third interval. Notice that the time trials in this session are accomplished in a bigger gear and with increasing heart-rate levels compared with sessions 8 and 11. The athlete is "dialing" the optimal gear, and learning or willing to work harder.
- The physiologic max heart rate for this rider is about 190. The session maximum heart rate was 185, over 97% of max.
- During the 3- and 4-minute time trials, heart rate rises rapidly to over 160 bpm, or about 85% of max.

Master Your Jump/Workout #12

Time	Gear	RPM		MPH
00:00	Easy	60		12
01:00		70		14
02:00		75		15
03:00		80		16
04:00		85		17
05:00		90		18
06:00		95		19
07:00		100		20
08:00		105		21
09:00		110		22
10:00		115		23
11:00		120		24
12:00		125		25
13:00				
14:00				
15:00				
16:00	52/17	80+		
17:00		140+		35 strokes or 15 sec. Count
18:00		140+		your strokes and set goals.
19:00		140+		
20:00		140+		
21:00		140+		
22:00		140+		
23:00		140+		
24:00		140+		30-sec sprint.
25:00	HR	HR		
26:00	HR	HR	HR	
27:00				
28:00				
29:00				
30:00	52/16	85		Should be a hard-gear effort.
31:00		85		4-min TT.
32:00		85		
33:00		85		
34:00	Rest			
35:00				
36:00	52/16	85		Should be a hard-gear effort.
37:00		85		4-min TT.
38:00		85		
39:00		85		
40:00	Rest			
41:00				
42:00	52/15	85		Should be a hard-gear effort.
43:00		85		3-min TT.
44:00		85		
45:00	HR	HR		
46:00	HR	HR	HR	
47:00				
48:00	42/17	80		
49:00		100		
50:00		125		
51:00		125		
52:00		125		
53:00		125		
54:00		100	110	
55:00		115	120	
56:00		125	130	
57:00		135	140+	
58:00	HR	HR		
59:00	HR	HR	HR	

Figure 12–31

Workout #12	Day		Date	
Format	12th Coached Trainer Session			
	Spin, Sprints, Intervals			

15 min	Warm-up	42/17	60–125	
10 min	Jumps	52/17	140+	
4 min	Interval	52/16	80–90	
4 min	Interval	52/16	80–90	
3 min	Interval	52/16	80–90	
7 min	Spin	42/17	to 125	
3 min	Spin-up	42/17	to 140	5rpm q30″

Seconds	0″	30″	60″	90″	120″
Last 30″ interval					
End of 3′ TT					
140 rpm					

Figure 12–32

JUMPS

Jumps are to be done in a gear that provides some resistance. After a minute in this gear, jump hard up to speed, and hold that fast cadence for 15 seconds. It may help to count your strokes. If you can achieve 140 rpm you'll get 35 strokes in 15 seconds.

Try to maintain or increase the number of strokes you achieve with each repetition. Perform a 15-second jump every minute for four repetitions. The last four jumps are for a variable period of time, from 5 to 30 seconds. Again, have someone tell you when to start and when to stop. You should perform each jump as if it will be for only 5 seconds. When the effort lasts longer, you will be very tired, having anticipated a much shorter effort. You will get much fitter!

TIME-TRIAL INTERVALS

Intervals of 3 to 4 minutes are done in the hardest gear you can push to complete the interval and maintain a cadence of 70–95. This depends upon your trainer, settings, preferences, and proclivities. HR readings should be 90% or more of max.

READ ACCOMPANYING HEART-RATE GRAPH

As in workouts 5, 8, and 11 I have provided a heart-rate graph to be used for comparison.

WORK ON FORM

With each time-trial interval concentrate on a different aspect of your form. For example, focus on pulling up, or keeping your knees in toward the top tube, or your back flat, or your elbows in, or your upper body relaxed, or your breathing rhythm. Work on technique and you'll go faster!

ASSESS, PLAN, ORGANIZE

We're at the end of the Trainer Series. It's time to review your goals for the upcoming season and reassess your strengths and weaknesses. It's time to plan for those few special events, whether it be your first competitive time trial or travel to Nationals. Set aside a few hours this weekend and plan the rest of your racing season. Also, use the next chapter's theme workouts to help you concentrate on working specific weaknesses or polishing fitness.

CHAPTER 13

Theme Workouts

The following nine stationary trainer workouts are designed to help you work on a particular aspect of fitness, whether it be leg strength, leg speed, aerobic capacity or anaerobic power. Whether you wish to improve leg speed with a spin workout or work on time trialing or hills, there is a workout designed for that specific aspect of fitness. There are even suggestions for a recovery workout in the easy-day workout.

The workouts in this series are as a group more difficult than the early workouts in the 12-Week Progressive Workout Series. If you are new to stationary training, you may wish to start with the 12-week series first.

Spin Workout

Time	Gear	Beginner RPM		Experienced RPM	
00:00	Warm-up	60		60	65
01:00	42/17	65		70	75
02:00	Easy	70		80	85
03:00		75		90	95
04:00		80		100	
05:00		85		105	
06:00		90		110	
07:00		95		115	
08:00				120	
09:00					
10:00		75		80	85
11:00		80		90	95
12:00		85		100	
13:00		90		105	
14:00		95		110	
15:00		100		115	
16:00		105		120	
17:00		110		125	
18:00				130	
19:00					
20:00		90		90	95
21:00		95		100	105
22:00		100		110	
23:00		105		115	
24:00		110		120	
25:00		115		125	
26:00		120		130	
27:00		125		135	
28:00				140	
29:00					
30:00		90			
31:00		95			
32:00		100			
33:00		105			
34:00		110		100	
35:00		115		100	
36:00		120	125	100	
37:00		130	135	100	
38:00				110	
39:00				110	
40:00		95		110	
41:00		95		110	
42:00		95		115	
43:00		95		115	
44:00		95		115	
45:00		100		115	
46:00		100		120	
47:00		100		120	
48:00		100		120	
49:00		100		120	
50:00	Cool-down				
51:00	42/17				
52:00		80		80	
53:00		90		90	
54:00		100		100	
55:00		100		100	
56:00		90		90	
57:00		80		80	
58:00		70		70	
59:00		60		60	

Figure 13–1

Spin Workout		Day		Date		
10 min	Warm-up	42/17				
8–9 min	Spin-up	42/17	2–3 ×			
10–16 min	Spin	42/17				
10 min	Cool-down	42/17				
Seconds		0″	30″	60″	90″	120″

Figure 13–2

PURPOSE
This session is designed to help you improve your spin. It will not help endurance but it may help your aerobic capacity.

BEGINNERS AND EXPERIENCED
I have charted two workouts, one for beginners with modest spin, and one for more experienced riders with good spin. These options are suggestions. Excellent spinners may increase all rpm by 20. After you perform this exercise a few times you will be able to easily tailor it to your level.

WARM-UP
Begin with a 10-minute warm-up. In an easy gear, progressively increase your rpm by 5 every minute until you can no longer increase them, or you have reached about 120 rpm. Once you develop good spin and leg speed, choosing a slightly harder gear while trying to maintain rpm goals will help develop your aerobic capacity.

SPIN-UPS
Perform two or three more spin-up repetitions. Once you can achieve a target rpm at the end of your last rep, and feel you could spin a little faster, begin the spin-ups at a higher rpm next workout.

SPIN
Spin for 10–16 minutes at a high rpm. Inch up as the exercise continues. Choose an rpm range just low enough that will allow you to complete the exercise. The range of rpm during this exercise should be no more than 20 rpm.

COOL-DOWN
Don't forget to cool down. Shift to an easy gear. Perform a spinning pyramid. Spin up to about 100 rpm, and then wind down.

After you have finished this workout, if you lie down and close your eyes, it might seem that your legs are still going around in circles.

Sprint Workout

Time	Gear	RPM			
00:00	Warm-up	60			
01:00	42/17	70			
02:00	Easy	75			
03:00		80			
04:00		85			
05:00		90			
06:00		95			
07:00		100			
08:00		105			
09:00		110			
10:00		115			
11:00		120			
12:00					
13:00					
14:00					
15:00	52/17	140+	Sprint	Sit	Drops
16:00	Moderate				
17:00			Sprint	Sit	Hoods
18:00					
19:00			Sprint	Sit	Drops
20:00					
21:00			Sprint	Sit	Hoods
22:00					
23:00					
24:00			Sprint	Stand	Drops
25:00					
26:00			Sprint	Stand	Hoods
27:00					
28:00			Sprint	Stand	Drops
29:00					
30:00			Sprint	Stand	Hoods
31:00					
32:00					
33:00			Sprint	Sit	Drops
34:00					
35:00			Sprint	Sit	Hoods
36:00					
37:00			Sprint	Sit	Drops
38:00					
39:00			Sprint	Sit	Hoods
40:00					
41:00					
42:00			Sprint	Stand	Drops
43:00					
44:00			Sprint	Stand	Hoods
45:00					
46:00			Sprint	Stand	Drops
47:00					
48:00			Sprint	Stand	Hoods
49:00					
50:00	Cool-down	60			
51:00	42/17	70			
52:00		80			
53:00		90			
54:00		100			
55:00		110			
56:00		100			
57:00		90			
58:00		70			
59:00		60			

Figure 13–3

Sprint Workout		Day			Date	
15 min	Warm-up	42/17				
16–35 min	Sprint	52/17	140		4q2' × 2–4 sets	
10 min	Cool-down	42/17				
Seconds		0″	30″	60″	90″	120″

Figure 13–4

PURPOSE
This session is designed to help you improve your sprint or leg speed. It will not help endurance or your aerobic capacity. It will, however, help your short-term energy production, the creatine phosphate system.

WARM-UP
Begin with the usual 15-minute warm-up. In an easy gear, progressively increase your rpm by 5 every minute until you can no longer increase them, or you have reached about 120 rpm.

BEGINNERS AND EXPERIENCED
If you are a beginner, perform only every second sprint, for a total of 8 sprints. If you are more experienced, you may perform 16 sprints. If you perform all 16 sprints, do them in sets of four, with an extra minute of recovery between sets.

At the beginning of every designated minute, sprint for 15 seconds, or about 35 pedal strokes. Continue to pedal without much effort between sprints.

GEAR SELECTION
Choose a gear easy enough to allow you to achieve a cadence of at least 120 rpm. Most of the time you are looking for a target cadence closer to 140. Some of the time you may want a gear that will allow you to pedal even faster. When you are a racer and have good leg speed, you should be able to spin at over 200 rpm for very short periods of time.

Choosing an easier gear that allows maximum rpm will improve your leg speed. Choosing a slightly harder gear may help with the initial power section, the jump, that begins the sprint.

VARY POSITION
Vary your position. Perform half of the sprints while seated, half while standing. Perform half of the sprints with your hands in the drops, half with your hands on the hoods. The idea is to train all the slightly different muscle groups involved in sudden accelerations.

COOL-DOWN
Don't forget to cool down. Shift to an easy gear. Perform a spinning pyramid. Spin up to about 110 rpm, and then wind down.

Aerobic Workout

Time	Gear	RPM	
00:00	Warm-up	60	
01:00	42/17	70	
02:00	Easy	75	
03:00		80	
04:00		85	
05:00		90	
06:00		95	
07:00		100	
08:00		105	
09:00		110	
10:00		115	
11:00		120	
12:00			
13:00			
14:00			
15:00	52/15	55	Stand, raise 4 in.
16:00	Moderate	55	
17:00	Hard	80	First 15 sec. only
18:00		80	"
19:00		80	"
20:00		80	"
21:00		80	"
22:00	Rest		
23:00			
24:00			
25:00	52/16	85	Hard 4-min TT.
26:00		85	
27:00		85	
28:00		85	
29:00	Rest		
30:00	52/16	85	Hard 4-min TT.
31:00		85	
32:00		85	
33:00		85	
34:00	Rest		
35:00			
36:00	42/16	110	
37:00		110	
38:00		110	
39:00		110	
40:00		110	
41:00		110	
42:00		110	
43:00		110	
44:00		110	
45:00		110	
46:00		110	
47:00	Rest	110	
48:00		110	
49:00		110	
50:00	Cool-down	60	
51:00	42/17	70	
52:00		80	
53:00		90	
54:00		100	
55:00		100	
56:00		90	
57:00		80	
58:00		70	
59:00		60	

Figure 13–5

Aerobic Workout		Day			Date		
15 min	Warm-up	42/17					
7 min	Stand	52/15	55–80		5 jumps		
4 min	Interval	52/16	85		2×		
10 min	Spin	42/16	110				
10 min	Cool-down	42/17					
Seconds		0″	30″	60″	90″	120″	

Figure 13–6

PURPOSE
This session is designed to help you improve aerobic capacity. To a modest extent it will also help strength, hill climbing, and spin.

WARM-UP
Begin with the usual 15-minute warm-up. In an easy gear, progressively increase your rpm by 5 every minute until you can no longer increase them, or you have reached about 120 rpm.

ELEVATE TRAINER
Elevate the front of your trainer on a block of wood. Raise it about 4 inches.

STAND
Stand in a moderately hard gear. After 2 minutes, jump up to 80 rpm for about 15 seconds. Partially recover as your cadence drops to 55 again for 45 seconds. Repeat at the top of each minute for a total of five 15-second accelerations.

Climbing and short efforts of this type are one of the quickest ways to raise your heart rate. Read about aerobic training in Chapter 10. After two accelerations your heart rate should be about 80% of your physiological maximum, and after the last effort it should be 85–90% of your max.

TIME-TRIAL INTERVALS
Level the bicycle and perform two 4-minute time trials in as hard a gear as you can push at about 85 rpm to just complete each interval.

SPIN
After a couple of minutes of recovery, shift to a moderately easy gear and spin 110 rpm (average) for 10 minutes. You may be 5–10 rpm lower the first few minutes. If you are not winded at the end of the 10 minutes, choose a harder gear next time.

COOL-DOWN
Don't forget to cool down. Shift to an easy gear. Perform a spinning pyramid. Spin up to about 100 rpm, and then wind down.

Hill Climbing Workout

Time	Gear	RPM	
00:00	Warm-up	60	
01:00	42/17	70	
02:00	Easy	75	
03:00		80	
04:00		85	
05:00		90	
06:00		95	
07:00		100	
08:00		105	
09:00		110	
10:00		115	
11:00		120	
12:00			
13:00			
14:00			
15:00	52/12	50–60	Stand, raise 4 in.
16:00	Hard		
17:00			
18:00			
19:00			
20:00			
21:00			
22:00			
23:00			
24:00			
25:00	52/13		Sit.
26:00			
27:00			
28:00			
29:00			
30:00	52/12	50–60	Stand, raise 6 in.
31:00			
32:00			
33:00			
34:00			
35:00			Sit.
36:00			
37:00			
38:00			
39:00			
40:00	52/12		Stand, raise 4 in.
41:00		60+	Sprint.
42:00		60	Sprint.
43:00		60	Sprint.
44:00			
45:00	52/13		Sit.
46:00		70+	Sprint.
47:00		70	Sprint.
48:00		70	Sprint.
49:00			
50:00	Cool-down	60	
51:00	42/17	70	
52:00		80	
53:00		90	
54:00		100	
55:00		110	
56:00		105	
57:00		80	
58:00		70	
59:00		60	

Figure 13–7

Hill Climbing Workout		Day		Date		
15 min	Warm-up	42/17				
10 min	Stand, 4 in.	52/12	50–60			
5 min	Sit, 4 in.	52/13	50–60			
5 min	Stand, 6 in.	52/12	50–60			
5 min	Sit, 6 in.	52/12	50–60			
4 min	Stand, 4 in.	52/12	60+	3 sprints		
4 min	Sit	52/13	70+	3 sprints		
10 min	Cool-down	42/17				
Seconds		0″	30″	60″	90″	120″

Figure 13–8

PURPOSE

This session is designed to help you improve hill climbing. It will help your strength and your aerobic ability but will not help spin.

WARM-UP

Begin with the usual 15-minute warm-up. In an easy gear, progressively increase your rpm by 5 every minute until you can no longer increase them, or you have reached about 120 rpm.

ELEVATE TRAINER

Elevate the front of your trainer on a block of wood, raising it about 4 inches.

STAND

Stand up on the trainer. In a very heavy gear turn the cranks at between 50 and 60 rpm. Spend time concentrating on pulling up as well as pushing down.

Beginners may wish to stand for only a few minutes. More experienced climbers can stand 10 minutes, and then sit down and push a slightly easier gear for 5 more minutes.

ELEVATE HIGHER

Recover, and raise the trainer to a total of 6 inches. In a very heavy gear, stand again for 5 minutes.

SIT

Sit for 5 minutes without shifting to an easier gear. If your trainer is not stable at this height, be careful you don't wheelie backward.

Recover.

HILL SPRINTS

Reduce your incline to 4 inches. While standing, sprint to over 60 rpm for the first 15 seconds of every minute over the course of 3 minutes. Sit down, recover for a full minute, and in a slightly easier gear perform three more sprints to at least 70 rpm. If you can achieve significantly more rpm than outlined, you have performed this exercise in too easy a gear.

COOL-DOWN

Don't forget to cool down. Shift to an easy gear. Perform a spinning pyramid. Spin up to about 110 rpm, and then wind down.

Easy Day Workout

Time	Gear	RPM	
00:00	Warm-up	60	
01:00	42/17	70	
02:00	Easy	75	
03:00		80	
04:00		85	
05:00		90	
06:00		95	
07:00		100	
08:00		105	
09:00		110	
10:00		115	
11:00		120	
12:00			
13:00			
14:00			
15:00	52/17	85	Read.
16:00	Moderate		
17:00			
18:00			Listen to music.
19:00			
20:00			
21:00			Talk on the phone.
22:00			
23:00			
24:00			Watch TV.
25:00			
26:00			
27:00			
28:00			
29:00			
30:00	52/17	50	Left leg ILT
31:00			
32:00			
33:00			Right leg ILT
34:00			
35:00			
36:00			
37:00			
38:00			
39:00			
40:00	52/17	85	Concentrate on position.
41:00			
42:00			
43:00			
44:00			
45:00			
46:00			
47:00			
48:00			
49:00			
50:00	Cool-down	60	
51:00	42/17	70	
52:00		80	
53:00		90	
54:00		100	
55:00		100	
56:00		90	
57:00		80	
58:00		70	
59:00		60	

Figure 13–9

Easy-Day Workout		Day		Date		
15 min	Warm-up	42/17				
15 min	Various	52/17	85			
6 min	ILT	52/17	50			
10 min	Position	52/17	85			
10 min	Cool-down	42/17				
Seconds		0"	30"	60"	90"	120"

Figure 13–10

PURPOSE

This session is designed to help you recover. It is not meant to train any specific area. It is meant as a rest day of active recovery.

Remember, most of us work too hard on our easy days, and not hard enough on our hard days.

WARM-UP

Begin with the usual 15-minute warm-up. In an easy gear, progressively increase your rpm by 5 every minute until you can no longer increase them, or you have reached about 120 rpm.

BE DISTRACTED

Find a copy of your favorite bicycling magazine. In a moderate gear, but without really thinking or worrying about it, pedal as you read an interesting article. Get your cordless phone or one with a long extension cord, if your trainer is not too noisy. Yak and gossip. Watch TV or listen to music. Accelerate your rpm if you feel like it whenever a commercial comes on, or the beat increases.

EASY ILT

Perform a little easy ILT. Don't worry about pushing a heavy gear, as when you are really trying to work on strength. Just let the legs go around.

THINK ABOUT FORM

Spend time concentrating on some aspect of position. Thinking about lowering your stem for time trialing? Pedal in the aero position with your stem lowered a little. Want to raise your seat a bit? Let your body adapt to position without any strain or concern about effort. Have a new pair of shoes? Break them in with easy riding while you figure out the best position for your cleats.

COOL-DOWN

Enjoy an easy cool-down. Shift to an easy gear. Perform a spinning pyramid. Spin up to about 100 rpm, and then wind down.

Enjoy your easy day. You deserve it. And you need it if you want to work hard later.

Criterium Workout

Time	Gear	Beginner RPM		Experienced RPM	
00:00	Warm-up	60		60	
01:00	42/17	70		70	
02:00	Easy	75		75	
03:00		80		80	
04:00		85		85	
05:00		90		90	
06:00		95		95	
07:00		100		100	
08:00		105		105	
09:00		110		110	
10:00		115		115	
11:00		120		120	
12:00					
13:00					
14:00	52/17	100		100	
15:00	Moderate	120		120	120
16:00		120		120	120
17:00		120		120	120
18:00		120		120	120
19:00		120		120	120
20:00					
21:00					
22:00					
23:00		120		120	120
24:00		120		120	120
25:00		120		120	120
26:00		120		120	120
27:00		120		120	120
28:00		120		120	120
29:00		120		120	120
30:00					
31:00					
32:00					
33:00				120	120
34:00				120	120
35:00		120		120	120
36:00		120		120	120
37:00		120		120	120
38:00		100		120	120
39:00		120	120	120	120
40:00		120	120	100	
41:00		120	120	120	120
42:00		120	120	120	120
43:00		120	120	120	120
44:00		120	120	120	120
45:00		120	120	120	120
46:00				120	120
47:00					
48:00					
49:00					
50:00	Cool-down	60		60	
51:00	42/17	70		70	
52:00		80		80	
53:00		90		90	
54:00		100		100	
55:00		100		100	
56:00		90		90	
57:00		80		80	
58:00		70		70	
59:00		60		60	

Figure 13–11

Criterium Workout		Day		Date		
15 min	Warm-up	42/17				
6 min	Jumps	52/17	120	5–10		
8 min	Jumps	52/17	120	7–14		
10–15 min	Jumps	52/17	120	17–26		
10 min	Cool-down	42/17				
Seconds		0″	30″	60″	90″	120″

Figure 13–12

PURPOSE
This session is designed to help you improve criterium riding. It will help your jump, your aerobic ability, your anaerobic threshold, and your sprint. It does not emphasize strength.

WARM-UP
Begin with the usual 15-minute warm-up. In an easy gear, progressively increase your rpm by 5 every minute until you can no longer increase them, or you have reached about 120 rpm.

BEGINNERS AND EXPERIENCED
I have charted two workouts—one for beginning racers, and one for more experienced racers. Criteriums are ridden by racers, not riders. This is a very demanding workout.

GEAR SELECTION
Choose a moderate gear. Only after having performed this exercise a few times will you know exactly which gear to choose. The optimal gear is the one that brings you to your anaerobic threshold. Toward the end of the workout, each jump should bring you just over your anaerobic threshold, and each partial recovery in between jumps should allow your heart rate to fall just below your threshold.

MAINTAIN RPM BETWEEN JUMPS
Always maintain at least 100 rpm between jumps. After riding at 100 rpm for 1 minute, jump to 120 rpm. You do not need to hold this faster cadence for any period of time. You have only to reach it momentarily.

JUMP AT LEAST EVERY MINUTE
Beginners do this once at the top of the minute for 5 jumps.

Experienced racers jump every 30 seconds for a total of 10 jumps.

After a few minutes of easy pedaling, perform a similar exercise. This time beginners perform 7 jumps, experienced racers 14.

Recover.

Beginners now jump 3 times, have an extra minute at 100 rpm, and then try jumping every 30 seconds for a total of 14 more jumps.

Experienced racers perform 14 jumps, have an extra minute of relative recovery at 100 rpm, and then perform 12 more jumps.

COOL-DOWN
Don't forget to cool down. Shift to an easy gear. Perform a spinning pyramid. Spin up to about 100 rpm, and then wind down.

Strength Workout

Time	Gear	RPM	
00:00	Warm-up	60	
01:00	42/17	70	
02:00	Easy	75	
03:00		80	
04:00		85	
05:00		90	
06:00		95	
07:00		100	
08:00		105	
09:00		110	
10:00		115	
11:00		120	
12:00			
13:00			
14:00			
15:00	52/15	55	Left leg ILT
16:00		55	
17:00		55	
18:00		55	
19:00			
20:00	52/15	55	Right leg ILT
21:00		55	
22:00		55	
23:00		55	
24:00			
25:00	52/14	50	Left leg ILT
26:00		50	
27:00		50	
28:00			
29:00	52/14	50	Right leg ILT
30:00		50	
31:00		50	
32:00			
33:00			
34:00	52/12	50	Stand, raise 4 in.
35:00		50	
36:00		50	
37:00		50	
38:00		50	
39:00		50	
40:00		50	
41:00		50	
42:00		50	
43:00		50	
44:00			
45:00		50	Sit.
46:00		50	
47:00		50	
48:00		50	
49:00		50	
50:00	Cool-down		
51:00	42/17	60	
52:00		70	
53:00		80	
54:00		90	
55:00		100	
56:00		110	
57:00		90	
58:00		70	
59:00		60	

Figure 13–13

Strength Workout		Day			Date	
15 min	Warm-up	42/17				
4 min	ILT	52/15	55			
3 min	ILT	52/14	50			
10 min	Stand, 4 in.	52/12	50			
5 min	Sit	52/12	50			
10 min	Cool-down	42/17				
Seconds		0″	30″	60″	90″	120″

Figure 13–14

PURPOSE

This session is designed to help you improve your strength. The second half hour may help develop your aerobic capacity.

WARM-UP

Begin with the usual 15-minute warm-up. In an easy gear, progressively increase your rpm by 5 every minute until you can no longer increase them, or you have reached about 120 rpm.

ISOLATED-LEG TRAINING

Spend 4 minutes with each leg performing isolated-leg training. Push a heavy gear at about 55 rpm. Then spend 3 minutes in a very heavy gear, the heaviest gear you can manage, pushing 50 rpm for 3 minutes.

HILL CLIMBING

Elevate the front of your trainer on a block of wood, raising it about 4 inches.

In a very heavy gear, stand and turn the cranks at about 50 rpm. Spend time concentrating on different parts of the stroke. Sometimes concentrate on pushing down, sometimes on pulling up.

SEATED PUSHING

After 10 minutes, sit down. Keep the front of the bike elevated. Continue to push a monster gear at about 50 rpm. Spend some time concentrating on pushing forward, rather than down.

COOL-DOWN

Don't forget to cool down. Shift to an easy gear. With the front of the bike still elevated, or with the bicycle position returned to level, perform a spinning pyramid. Spin up to about 110 rpm, and then wind down.

Isolated-Leg Training Workout

Time	Gear	RPM		
00:00	Warm-up	60		
01:00	42/17	70		
02:00	Easy	75		
03:00		80		
04:00		85		
05:00		90		
06:00		95		
07:00		100		
08:00		105		
09:00		110		
10:00		115		
11:00		120		
12:00				
13:00				
14:00				
15:00	52/15	55	Left leg ILT	
16:00		55		
17:00		55		
18:00	Rest			
19:00	52/15	55	Right leg ILT	
20:00		55		
21:00		55		
22:00	Rest			
23:00	52/14	50	Left leg ILT	
24:00		50		
25:00		50		
26:00		50		
27:00	Rest			
28:00	52/14	50	Right leg ILT	
29:00		50		
30:00		50		
31:00		50		
32:00	Rest			
33:00	52/14	50	Left	
34:00		50		
35:00		50		
36:00	Rest			
37:00	52/14	50	Right	
38:00		50		
39:00		50		
40:00	Rest			
41:00	52/15	50	Left	
42:00		60+		Sprint
43:00		60+		Sprint
44:00		60+	Right	Sprint
45:00		60+		Sprint
46:00		50	Left	
47:00		60+		Sprint
48:00		60+		Sprint
49:00		60+	Right	Sprint
50:00		60+		Sprint
51:00	Cool-down			
52:00	42/17	70		
53:00		80		
54:00		90		
55:00		100		
56:00		110		
57:00		90		
58:00		70		
59:00		60		

Figure 13–15

Isolated-Leg Training Workout		Day		Date		
15 min	Warm-up	42/17				
3 min	ILT	52/15	55			
4 min	ILT	52/14	50			
3 min	ILT	52/14	50			
4 min	ILT	52/15	60+	10″ q1′		
10 min	Cool-down	42/17				
Seconds	0″	30″	60″	90″	120″	

Figure 13–16

PURPOSE
This session is designed to improve strength and power. It will not help your aerobic capacity.

WARM-UP
Begin with the usual 15-minute warm-up. In an easy gear, progressively increase your rpm by 5 every minute until you can no longer increase them, or you have reached about 120 rpm.

ILT SETS
Spend 3 minutes with each leg performing isolated leg training. Push a heavy gear at about 55 rpm.

Continue to turn the cranks during the rest minutes. This may help to prevent cramping and promote recovery for the next repetition.

Shift to the hardest gear you can push at a cadence of about 50 rpm. Perform 4 minutes of isolated-leg training with each leg.

After a minute of rest, repeat this exercise for 3 minutes with each leg.

POSITION SPECIFICITY
If you wish to improve your time trialing, perform ILT with aerobars in your time-trial position. If you wish to improve your hill climbing, perform ILT with the front of your trainer raised 4 inches and your hands on the tops.

CONCENTRATE ON SECTIONS OF YOUR STROKE
Concentrate on different sections of your stroke. Some of the time concentrate on pushing down, some of the time on pulling up or pushing forward.

ILT SPRINTS
Rest a minute or two. Shift to a slightly easier gear.

After a minute of ILT, sprint with one leg as hard as you can for 10 seconds. Do another sprint a minute later. Switch legs during the 50-second recovery, and do two sprints with your other leg.

Allow an extra minute of recovery, then repeat the exercise—two sprints with each leg. This makes a total of eight ILT sprints.

Beginners might be happy with a total of four ILT sprints.

COOL-DOWN
Don't forget to cool down. Shift to an easy gear. Perform a spinning pyramid. Spin up to about 100 rpm, and then wind down.

Time-Trial Workout

Time	Gear	RPM	
00:00	Warm-up	60	
01:00	42/17	70	
02:00	Easy	75	
03:00		80	
04:00		85	
05:00		90	
06:00		95	
07:00		100	
08:00		105	
09:00		110	
10:00		115	
11:00		120	
12:00			
13:00			
14:00			
15:00	52/15	55	Left leg ILT
16:00	Moderate	55	
17:00		55	
18:00		55	
19:00	Rest		
20:00	52/15	55	Right leg ILT
21:00		55	
22:00		55	
23:00		55	
24:00			
25:00	52/14	50	Left leg ILT
26:00		50	
27:00		50	
28:00			
29:00	52/14	50	Right leg ILT
30:00		50	
31:00		50	
32:00	Rest		
33:00			
34:00			
35:00	52/15	75–90	
36:00		75–90	
37:00		75–90	
38:00		75–90	
39:00		75–90	
40:00		75–90	
41:00		75–90	
42:00		75–90	
43:00		75–90	
44:00		75–90	
45:00		75–90	
46:00		75–90	
47:00		75–90	
48:00		75–90	
49:00		75–90	
50:00		75–90	
51:00		75–90	
52:00		75–90	
53:00		75–90	
54:00		75–90	
55:00	Cool-down		
56:00	42/17		
57:00			
58:00			
59:00			

Figure 13–17

Time-Trial Workout		Day		Date		
15 min	Warm-up	42/17				
4 min	ILT	52/15	55			
3 min	ILT	52/14	50			
20 min	TT	52/15	75–90			
5 min	Cool-down	42/17				
Seconds		0″	30″	60″	90″	120″

Figure 13–18

PURPOSE
This session is for those motivated to improve their time trialing. It is designed to provide some strength training, as well as anaerobic threshold work.

WARM-UP
Begin with the usual 15-minute warm-up. In an easy gear, progressively increase your rpm by 5 every minute until you can no longer increase them, or you have reached about 120 rpm.

POSITION
It is important to train specifically. Perform the ILT and the 20-minute time trial in your "aero" position. Ideally, you'll have the same setup on your trainer as on your TT bike—aerobars and position the same.

ILT INTERVALS
Spend 4 minutes with each leg performing isolated-leg training. Push a heavy gear at about 55 rpm. Then spend 3 minutes in a very heavy gear, the heaviest gear you can manage, pushing at 50 rpm for 3 minutes.

Rest for a few minutes.

20-MINUTE TIME TRIAL
Ride for 20 minutes at your time-trial cadence, pushing a hard gear to achieve a target heart rate of 85% or more of your max by the end of the effort. By observing your cadence monitor, aim to work uniformly throughout the 20 minutes. If you are able to increase your cadence in the last half by more than 5 rpm, try a heavier gear or a faster cadence at the start of your next time-trial workout.

LENGTH OF TIME TRIAL MAY VARY
If you are just beginning time-trial workouts, consider performing a shorter time trial, perhaps 10 minutes. If you are peaking toward a 40K event, consider dropping the first ILT repetition and increasing the length of your time trial to 25 or 30 minutes.

COOL-DOWN
Don't forget to cool down by spinning easily for at least 5 minutes.

Stationary Trainer Heart-Rate Graph: Time-Trial Workout

This is a recording of a fit athlete during a period of specialized time-trial training. The athlete has 5 days until Senior Nationals and 5 weeks until Masters Nationals. The primary goal of this session was anaerobic threshold training and leg strength.

THE WORKOUT
- Warm-up was performed in a relatively easy gear, spinning up from 60 to 120 rpm.
- 5 minutes of recovery.
- 4 minutes of isolated leg training for each leg, with 30 seconds between each leg.
- A few minutes of recovery.
- A 27-minute time trial pushing 76 rpm.

Figure 13–19 **Theme stationary trainer work: time-trial training.**

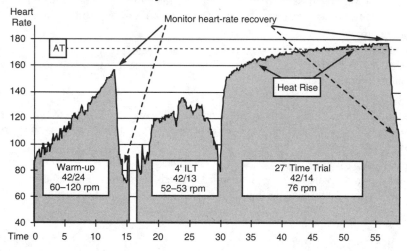

Notice:

- Heart rate rises predictably and smoothly with the warm-up.
- Isolated-leg training promotes leg strength, but is not an aerobic workout.
- The athlete rode the entire time trial at a cadence between 75 and 77 rpm. The effort is constant from 30 to 57 minutes. Rising heart rate from 30 to 57 minutes reflects rising body temperature.
- The time-trial section is aimed at power development. Leg strength and aerobic effort are both involved in this drill. Had this drill been conducted at a higher rpm, heart rate would have been higher.
- The physiologic maximum heart rate for this rider is 191. The session maximum heart rate was 177, or about 93% of max.
- The athlete spent about two-thirds of the time trial within five beats of his anaerobic threshold.
- Recovery is excellent.

Part Four

RACING

For those of you who want to become serious about racing, there is a lot you'll need to take in as you read the coming pages. If you have never raced before, you may not fully understand many of the concepts in this part of the book until you have actually experienced them first-hand. Don't despair! There is no substitute for experience and this part of the book is not meant to be consumed all at once. Come back to certain chapters when the need arises and always keep the basics in mind. To help you do that, here are a few hints.

- Don't try new equipment or foods for the first time in competition.
- Ride with groups just a little beyond your level.
- Ride with groups below your abilities to learn how to control, lead, and assert yourself in a group. It's a skill that's important but hard to learn when others are stronger than you.
- When your group is warming up or cooling down, ride in a smaller gear than just about everyone else to learn to spin better.
- Train strength by riding hills or into the wind in big gears at about 50 rpm.
- Learn to work hard on a stationary trainer. Join a class if that's what it takes.
- Work on your weaknesses in the off-season, work on your strengths in season.
- Practice sprints. Training this aspect of racing will put you ahead of the majority of racers who, unbelievably, never practice it!
- Practice skills such as bumping and touching wheels with others on a smooth, grassy field.
- Train in the drops—you'll better develop the muscles you use in racing and be faster. (Most riders tend to race in the drops, except when climbing. Train the same way. The reason you sometimes ride the hoods is because you get more power that way. The reason you race in the drops is because, at fast speeds, the better aerodynamics more than compensate for the reduced power and you go faster.)
- Don't ride steady. Learn to surge, jump, and see what happens when the group splits. Far too many club riders ride paceline far too often. Paceline is a skill you should have. It doesn't mean you should always train that way.
- Every use of energy should have a purpose. When you decide to use

your energy, especially to make a jump or move in a race, do so with commitment.

- Think not only about your own strategy and tactics: Consider what moves your opponents are likely to make to achieve their goals—plan accordingly.
- Watch the good riders and study how they flow without doing any more work than necessary. Try to learn from them.
- Upgrade by your placings, not experience. You may have raced in Category 4 for a long time and feel you are fit enough to upgrade, but how are your placings? Placings reflect not only your physical ability and experience but your skill level as well. By waiting and upgrading according to placings, you'll force yourself to become a better all-around rider.

CHAPTER 14

Racing Basics

It is easier to start racing with the right preparation and knowledge. Most of the information discussed below applies to United States Cycling Federation (USCF) racing, although information about mountain biking is also presented.

Types of Bicycle Races

Most well known are the Olympic-type races: those held on roadways, called road races; those on specialized tracks called velodromes; and those off-road, mountain biking.

The USCF is the U.S. amateur national governing body for road and track racing. Pro Cycling is the U.S. professional national governing body for road and track cycling. NORBA—the National Off-Road Bicycle Association—is the U.S. national governing body of mountain bike racing. USA Cycling is the umbrella organization for USCF, US Pro, and NORBA.

Other types of races include BMX (bicycle motor cross), mostly for younger riders; endurance events such as the Race Across AMerica (RAAM); and HPV (human-powered vehicle) races, where bicycles may use fairings.

Races may be individual competitions against the clock for time, called time trials, or events where many riders start together, called mass-start races. Time trials are discussed in detail in Chapter 19.

ROAD RACES

Road races are of several types: time trials, criteriums, and road races.

- Time trials are races against the clock; you ride by yourself over a distance for time. Such races are typically held for 10 miles at the local level, or 40K (a little under 25 miles) at the state or national level.
- Criteriums are races on circuits up to a mile in length, often with many corners, and frequently on flat terrain. These races involve specific racing skills such as cornering and riding together in close groups (packs). The ability to surge and respond to differences in speed quickly is important in these events.
- Road races are typically held over smaller state highways or partially closed urban routes. These are more like the rides most beginning cyclists may be familiar with, only at speed.

TRACK RACES

Track races involve many different types of racing. The traditional championship events are sprints, points races, and time-trial-like events over distances of 1, 3, or 4 kilometers (about 0.5 to about 2.5 miles). Weekly local velodrome racing has many more types of mass-start race formats than can be listed here.

- Sprint competitions are usually held over distances of about 0.5 mile. Two or three riders participate at a time. Because of the effect of the slipstream, the sprint often does not begin in earnest until only 200 meters (yards) are left in the race!
- Points races are over many laps—say, 50—with mini-competitions—say, every 5 laps. Points are awarded to the lead four riders of each mini-competition. Final placings are determined from the overall winners of the mini-races.
- Kilos or 1-kilometer time trials are individual races for that distance on the track.
- Pursuits are races over 3 or 4 kilometers. For most riders these competitions are events with an opponent on the opposite side of the track, performed in heats. In masters racing, they are individual efforts for time.

MOUNTAIN BIKE RACES

Off-road or riding in the dirt is the newest and perhaps most popular type of racing. Normally raced on a circuit course, often with room for only one bicycle—single track—specialized forms of mountain biking include downhill, criterium style, and dual slalom.

Get Your Bike from a Bike Store

You have choices and considerations when selecting a bicycle. You'll need to decide price range, size, types of components, as well as color. You can purchase a bicycle through mail order, at department stores, or at specialty bicycle stores. The better specialty stores are known as "pro shops."

There is a tremendous selection available. Although mail order is at first glance less expensive, it may be a false savings. Service and competent advice are paramount. There is little point in investing upwards of $1,500 on a wonderful bicycle only to find out a few months later that it really is too large a fit.

Look for a pro bike shop that supports racers and racing. Such shops often advertise in local racing publications, support local bicycle racing clubs, or are found as technical support at local races.

How Many Miles Do You Need to Train?

Most road riders who race train at least 100 miles weekly. The norm for competitive riders in Categories 3, 4, and 5 is 150–250 miles a week.

Ride with Others, Join a Club

Look for a bicycling club oriented toward racing. If you are a masters rider, seek a club with a masters interest group. Juniors should look for juniors programs, and women should look for clubs that have a special interest in their development.

Most clubs will allow you to ride with them for several weeks at no charge. This will be a good time to assess your abilities, and to determine whether the club is suitable for you. If you enjoy riding with the club, you can usually join for about $35. There is no need to obtain a license to race in order to join a club.

Once you start riding with a group, you will learn a lot of things you really did not need to know when riding on your own: how to follow another rider closely, yet safely, to expend less effort; how to turn a corner without a loss in speed; how to suddenly and explosively accelerate your bicycle. These skills are required in racing, but not in solo riding.

Most clubs have training or development races, in which you can ease your way into a race atmosphere without formally entering a licensed race. Such training races will give you a good idea of what is required to race. You can judge yourself against the already established racers and find out at what level you are riding.

Please don't be too intimidated by the racers and their somewhat cliquish behavior. They all wear those black shorts and fancy jerseys, and seem to know everything. Sometimes they act a little weird. Frequently they are worried about a new rider riding in an unpredictable way, and they translate their anxieties into rude shouts and yells. Remember, those racers started out just like you, and had many skills to learn!

Ideally the club you have selected will have a beginners group, where experienced racers and coaches will show you the ropes and teach racing safety and skills.

Starting with Time Trials

Few special skills are required to race by yourself against the clock. For this reason time trials are a good way to see how you are doing and assess your prospects for racing with others (mass-start races).

Men aged 19 to 29: If you can ride 10 miles in under 30 minutes you may be ready for mass-start racing. Women, older masters, and juniors: Add a couple of minutes.

Starting Mass-Start Racing

Bicycling is very different from jogging or running. Whereas anyone can go out and run, bicycle racing involves considerably more skill.

If you go out to run a 10K, chances are some runners will be a lot slower and some a lot faster. You can continue to train on your own, and strive to improve your personal 10K time. When you start a bicycle race with others, however, a prerequisite level of ability is required, because you must be able to stay with the main group of riders (the pack). Without the benefit of the pack's slipstream breaking air resistance, you are out of the race.

The slipstream is much less important in most mountain biking, where speeds are slower. Skill and time-trialing ability are more important.

Most races require you to have a racing license, although you may occasionally see one advertised as a public or citizen race where a license is not required. This might be a place to start, but such races are infrequent.

Your First Course

For your first races choose a course without many sharp turns and without many challenging hills. In this way you will be more likely able to stay with the group and finish. As you see how you do, and judge your skills, you'll know better when to enter more challenging races.

After racing a few times, you'll want even more information on the specifics of training, intervals, sprint workouts, etc. Though often such information is available from books such as this one, your club will be in the best position to help you.

Track Racing

Is there a velodrome in your area? Many velodromes have development or interest courses to help.

Age and Sex Categories

Juniors are 18 years of age and under. Seniors are aged 19 to 29. Masters are 30 and over. Women usually race separately, sometimes all lumped into one group.

Ability Categories—Upgrading

Racers are categorized by experience and talent. In USCF racing there are five categories for amateur male riders, four for females. Men begin as Category 5 riders, women as Category 4. Category 1 is the top level of amateur rider.

It is possible to upgrade from Cat 5 to 4, or from Cat 4 to 3, based on experience or results. To upgrade from Cat 3 to Cat 2, or from Cat 2 to 1, results are required.

A points system assigns a certain number of points based on placing, more points being given for higher placings. A certain number of points makes it possible (or necessary) to upgrade.

Your district rep is responsible for upgrades. Your district rep's telephone number and upgrading requirements and procedures are listed in your rule book.

Masters Racing

About half of all racers in the United States are masters.

Masters racing starts at age 30, but the event promoter may choose to have a race for a specific age group—for example, those over 35 or 45.

You can race by age if you are a masters racer, or by category. If you are a 37-year-old male, it is sometimes more fun and safer to race with those over 35 years old. But you may have to race with all those over 35 years old, which may include some Cat 3 and Cat 2 riders. Or you may choose to race with the Cat 5's without age restriction. Or you may race both!

Women

Women always have the prerogative to race with men, but not vice versa. Some choose to race with men in order to train at a higher level. Masters women may race with masters men up to 20 years older than they are.

CHAPTER 15

Your First Race: Stuff to Know!

You've decided to enter your first race. Here are some of the basics you'll need to know to let you concentrate on racing!

Rule Book

Like any sport, cycling has rules and regulations to assure fair competition and the safety of participants. Each year the USCF publishes a rule book.

This book includes a schedule of fees, the articles of incorporation and bylaws of USA Cycling, the bylaws of the United States Cycling Federation, categorization guidelines, the rules of racing, a list of U.S.A. champions for the last 10 years, current USCF National and World Cycling records, and other information.

You should review this book thoroughly when you receive it.

Where to Find Out about Races

When you join the USCF you receive *Cycling USA,* a monthly magazine about racing. It lists important regional and national races, but it probably won't help you find local races.

Many districts have local racing associations that publish listings of all races in the district.

Contact your local USCF district representative to inquire about local races. Your district rep's name and telephone number are in the back of the USCF rule book.

Ask your local bicycle racing club how to find out about local races.

Registration

There are two possibilities: You may register for a race the day of the race, or you may preregister.

For some races, entry is restricted to those who preregister. For other races, only day-of-the-race entry is available.

Local track racing usually has only day-of-the-race registration. Big important events often are by preregistration only.

Extremely popular races may be completely filled to capacity by preregistration and no day-of-the-race registration may be possible.

Multiple Entries

You may be able to enter more than one race at any given event, often at a reduced fee.

For example, a 37-year-old male, new to racing, might enter a Category 5 or a Masters 30–39 event.

A 37-year-old Cat 3 female might enter a Cat 3–4 women's event, a Cat 4–5 men's event (women may enter races categorized for men up to one category lower), or a masters men 45+ event (masters women may enter male masters races in age groups up to 20 years older).

The promoter chooses which categories of racing to offer. Junior racing, category racing for women, and 5-year masters racing are not always offered.

Field Limit

The number of racers that may enter a given race is restricted.

For Category 5 events, no more than 50 riders may enter. For other races, unless otherwise specifically restricted or noted, the field limit is 100 riders.

Attached/Unattached

To encourage membership in bicycling clubs that foster local racing, riders who do not race for recognized bicycle clubs often must pay a premium, or unattached fee.

Late Fee

When preregistration is available for a race, those who enter after a pre-registration deadline often pay a late fee.

Arriving at Your First Race

Plan on arriving at least 1 hour before your race is scheduled to start. Although races do run behind schedule, they are always on time when you are late.

You'll need time to get your numbers, locate the course, and warm up. For some events riders warm up for over 1 hour.

Locate the registration table. There may be a separate shorter line for those who have preregistered. Everyone has to show their racing license in order to race.

Determine from the officials present whether the race is running on schedule.

Check where numbers are to be placed, and pick up some safety pins. It's a good idea to have extra pins in your race bag—the promoter occasionally runs out.

Locate the portable toilets.

It's your responsibility to know the course. You'll want to be especially aware of the starting and finishing areas. For some races, you'll want to scout out the racecourse before race day.

Riders are usually called to the line at the start of a race. Occasionally they are called to a separate staging area before promenading to the start line. Determine if your race has a separate staging area.

Numbers

Numbers are necessary for officials to score races. Officials do not look to recognize riders when they assign placings—they look at numbers.

It is important that officials be able to read your numbers in order to determine your order of finish in a race.

Frequently only one number is given to riders. In many other events two are provided. In big, important races five numbers may be given—two for the back, two for the shoulders, and one for the bicycle. It is important to place your numbers correctly so that officials can easily read them.

Officials may be located on either side of the road. When only one number is given, you must determine on which side of the road the officials will be placed at the finish line, and pin your number accordingly.

When only one number is given, it is usually placed on the mid-back, on the same side as the side of the road where the finish-line officials will be, sideways, facing out.

Although some riders fold the empty, wide edges of their numbers and decrease the surface area of their number, the loss of contrast between black numbers and white background makes its harder for officials to read numbers. It is against the rules.

A trick to pinning on numbers nicely by yourself is to use your car's steering wheel to hold your jersey. Your number will be better attached if you avoid the corner holes and pin through and through the edges of the number.

Racing for Time/Racing for Laps

Criterium races can be raced over a certain distance or for a period of time. When raced for distance, the number of laps is specified before the race in the race announcement and by the official starting the race.

To help promoters keep their races on schedule, criterium races are sometimes raced for a certain period of time. For example, a criterium might be 45 minutes long. The officials make a determination of the average time it takes for riders to complete a lap. When the time left roughly equals the time it would take to complete, for example, five laps, the lap counter is brought into play on a countdown from five.

Mechanicals/Mishaps

There is a difference between an "unavoidable" problem with the bicycle and a lack of maintenance.

A mishap is a crash or mechanical accident (tire puncture or other failure of an essential component). A puncture caused by the sew-up tire coming off the rim owing to inadequate gluing is not considered a mechanical accident; neither is a malfunction due to misassembly or insufficient tightening of any component.

Make sure your bicycle is in tip-top shape before you race. Pumps and road kit bags should not be on a bicycle in a criterium.

Free Lap Rule

Flats, broken spokes, and other mechanical problems occasionally plague all riders. In criteriums, this sort of bad luck is often mitigated by the free lap rule, which allows riders suffering mishaps to fix their mechanical problems and reenter the race the next lap. You must make up lost distance in a road race, time trial, or criterium if no free lap rule is in effect.

Repairs must be made in a designated repair pit. Riders must proceed to the pit by continuing to travel along the course, in the direction of the race, until they arrive at the pit. If shortcuts to the pit are permitted, this will be announced by the starter before the race begins.

Riders suffering mishaps reenter the race at the back of the group of riders they were riding with before the mishap. If, for example, they were in the main group, they reenter the race at the back of that group. If they were in a breakaway, they may reenter the race in the breakaway.

Since the short rest that the free lap provides could give an unfair advantage near the end of a race, the free lap rule is not in effect in the last 8 kilometers of a race. This usually translates into five or six laps. Riders suffering mishaps are ineligible for primes for one lap after reentering the race.

If it is determined that the problem was foreseeable and due to a lack of reasonable maintenance of your bicycle, your problem may not be considered a mishap. You will have to make up lost ground and you will not be accorded a free lap.

Hand-ups in Road Races/Feeding

Riders often require more liquids or calories than they can conveniently carry to complete a race. Road races over 1 hour in length often have feed zones where riders may pick up additional liquid or food. Riders do not stop; they pick up these hand-ups while continuing to ride.

Occasionally the promoter will provide volunteers to assist riders at a neutral feed zone. Normally, you'll rely on a friend or teammate to assist you. Giving and receiving a hand-up requires some skill. Ask more experienced riders about their technique and practice with your feeder before the race.

For the safety of riders, the location of these feed zones is specified and predetermined; riders may pick up only in these areas. Normally, feeding is allowed only from the right side of the road.

The location of feeding zones is usually on a steady uphill grade. Downhill and level grades are unsuitable because the speed of riders is too great for safe pickups. Short climbs are often unsuitable because attacks and tactical racing frequently occur in these areas.

Regardless of their location, feed zones are often places where riders attack, although some consider it nonsporting to do so.

Role of Officials

In any race there are a number of uniformed, licensed officials. Depending upon the size of the race, one person may perform more than one duty. Not all race duties may be necessarily assigned to licensed officials.

- Chief referee: Supervises the general conduct of the race, interprets and enforces the rules, and makes rulings. May impose penalties for infractions. Decisions are final subject to a hearing for an appeal.
- Assistant referees: Advise the chief referee. May inspect bicycles and apparent mishaps.
- Judge and assistant judges: Determine the order of finish of a race.
- Scorers: Keep track of laps gained or lost by riders. Operate lap cards and bell.
- Timers: Compile times pertinent to classification.
- Starters: Call riders, inform riders of race distance and special rules governing race, inform riders of finish line if different from starting line. With the chief judge, assure riders' clothing, numbers, and equipment are proper. Judge whether a start is valid.
- Registrars: Confirm that entrants have valid racing licenses and are properly entered.

Checking Race Results

The number of places is announced before the start of the race. In an extremely small field only one rider may be recognized. Occasionally 50 riders in a large, national-level competition may be placed. In Category 3, 4, and 5 racing, normally 5 to 10 places are awarded.

Finished your race and think you've placed? Well maybe you have, and maybe you haven't. In the rush for the line, adrenaline sometimes clouds judgment and you may be mistaken as to where you thought you finished.

Occasionally the officials cannot place you. If your number was positioned so the officials could not read it, they may omit you from the placings.

Anyone can make a mistake. It's important to check the officials' results.

In races that are easy to score, results may be posted in just a few minutes. In others, where a finish requires close examination of a photograph, where many races are being held simultaneously, or where all participants' finishing times are individually recorded, results can take hours.

Once results are posted, you have 15 minutes to protest their validity. After 15 minutes, the posted results become official.

Protests and Appeals

A protest is a formal request by a rider or team manager to have a race official review a decision or oversight.

Protests regarding the qualification of riders or machines, the regularity of entries, or classifications should be lodged with the chief referee before the race.

In events consisting of a single race, protests regarding the order of finish or final results must be made within 15 minutes after the posting of results.

Protests of foul riding or other irregularity during a race must be made within 15 minutes after the protester's finish time.

An appeal is a formal request for review by an appeals jury of a suspension or qualification in a race.

After Your Race

The race is over. But your job isn't finished. There are still important things to do.

WHAT WE'RE TALKING ABOUT

It's a common scene. A rider finishes a race, and stands around chatting with friends and teammates for a couple of hours in the sun. Sounds innocent enough. But after a race there are a number of important things to do. Chatting in the sun may or may not be on the agenda.

RECOVER

Fluids and Energy Sources

Drink a bottle or two after your race—you are almost certainly dehydrated.

Eat something, too—replacing a few hundred calories of carbohydrates helps to quickly refuel your energy supplies.

If you are planning on training or racing again in the next few days, you've got to resupply your energy tanks.

You've heard of the glycogen tank and the glycogen window? Glycogen is the high-energy fuel of choice. You've got to get in a few hundred calories, preferably within the first half hour, to optimize the recharging of your glycogen tank. And then another few hundred more calories within another hour or two. At a minimum.

Do not wait hours for dinner—certainly have dinner later, but eat something ASAP.

Muscles

Those legs of yours have worked hard. Don't stand around for a couple of hours chatting or watching the next race. You can still be friendly and exchange war stories. But sit down to do it—get off your legs.

Crotch

Change out of those tight damp shorts. Biking shorts are great for biking—but the tightness and dampness are bad for crotch hygiene and promote saddle sores.

Thermal Stress

Heat increases the metabolic demands on the body. If it's a hot sunny day, and you stay exposed, you'll delay recovery. If you're not going home, get in the shade.

If it's cold or rainy, of course you'll want to get out of the weather and get into warm, dry clothes as soon as possible.

CHECK RACE RESULTS

Check the official results.

As mentioned, in races that are easy to score, results may be posted in just a few minutes. In others, results can take hours.

Once results are posted, you have 15 minutes to protest their validity; if there are no protests after 15 minutes, the posted results become official.

CONSIDER YOUR PERFORMANCE

In almost every race some things go well, others less than optimally. Consider in what ways you performed well; consider how you might improve.

Don't whine to others how you might have done better, how equipment problems prevented your win, how other riders teamed up against you, how it "wasn't your fault" you didn't do better. If you have a legitimate beef, protest quietly.

You might discuss equipment or tactical issues quietly with your mechanic, coach, or teammate. But such discussion should not be for public consumption.

PODIUM APPEARANCE?

You've placed or won. There's an etiquette of proper podium behavior. You'll see many riders who don't follow this etiquette. What can I say? There are lots of people who are rude, steal, or cheat. It doesn't make their behavior correct.

Appear for the Presentation

In big races the podium appearance is an important part of the total race presentation. In major tours, television exposure is an important financial asset for the promoter. Failure to appear for the podium presentation may result in a fine to the rider.

Some riders feel second place isn't worth anything—winning is all. I've raced with some riders who won't appear on the podium in second place. They just go home.

Sure, the races most of us do are small, and the presentations are often informal. Appear nonetheless. It's polite, it's proper etiquette, it's correct behavior—and it's just good manners.

Wear Your Current Club or Sponsors' Jersey

Your club or sponsors have supported you and have financially contributed to your racing. You are cheating them if you appear on the podium in a T-shirt, last year's jersey, or a torn or sloppy jersey.

You'll never see a Tour de France rider appear on the podium in anything other than the team jersey.

Some clubs that pay race support refuse to reimburse their riders for racing unless podium appearances have been made in the current club jersey.

There often isn't much the average beginning racer can do to help support the sponsors. Here's one way to do it: Wear your current club jersey.

Look Pleased

I've seen plenty of riders pleased to have finished a race with the field. Others have been disappointed because they have been pipped out of the win. I've seen riders in second place scowl and look dejected. Some occasionally refuse to shake the hands of their competitors on the podium.

In the big scheme of things, we're all lucky to be able to ride bikes and race. Looking pleased (and actually feeling pleased to participate) whether you're first or last is part of good sportsmanship.

THANK OTHERS

Give appropriate credit to others—teammates and other supporters—for your successes. Promoting a race takes a lot of time and energy. Make it a habit to thank at least one person—whether the promoter, a local sponsor, or corner-marshal volunteer—every race.

CHAPTER 16

Technique

Group Riding Principles

Certain principles apply when riding in a pack of riders. These principles are vital to the safety of the group and its members. Learn them and you'll be welcome in the paceline.

NO SUDDEN MOVES

Don't suddenly turn right, turn left, speed up, slow down. It is inefficient and dangerous.

BE SMOOTH

Riders new to pacelines feel the need to show they can keep up. Some work harder and speed up at the front. This is wrong. The front rider relinquishing the lead moves over to the side and then slows down, slightly. The rider assuming the lead does not speed up, but maintains the same speed.

GIVE OTHERS A TURN

The idea is not to prove how strong you are by hogging the front, but rather to learn how to work together in a group, ride together, and feel comfortable changing positions. There will be plenty of time to test your strength.

PULL OFF IN A CONSISTENT DIRECTION

When riding in a group, unless the wind changes, riders will relinquish the lead by "pulling off" to either the left or the right. Whichever way the group is working, pull off the same way.

DRAFT REASONABLY CLOSE

Keep as close to the rider in front of you as is comfortable and safe. Try not to let "gaps" open.

RIDE CLOSE SIDE TO SIDE

When you drop back to rotate, try to ride closely side by side as well. This is also much more efficient.

WARN OF ROAD HAZARDS

If there is plenty of time, everyone can avoid the hazard. If there is not much time to avoid some glass or a hole, it is often safer to ride over the hazard, rather than violate Rule 1—no sudden moves.

USE BRAKES AS LITTLE AS POSSIBLE

Braking wastes the energy you've used building up to speed. It is also dangerous for the rider in back of you.

DON'T EXHAUST YOURSELF BY PULLING TOO LONG

If you are weaker than the other riders in the group, take the front only for a few pedal strokes. Take your turn in front to practice technique and keep the paceline flowing smoothly.

DON'T FOOL WITH WATER BOTTLES OR FOOD WHEN LEADING

Wait until you've pulled off. Also, try to be in the correct gear and not change gears when you are leading.

DO NOT OVERLAP WHEELS

Ride behind the rider in front of you. With a crosswind, experienced racers ride partially to the side of the rider in front of them to help shield them from the wind. If the rider in front of you moves over slightly, and you are overlapping that back wheel, it is your front end that will be unstable, and it is you who will go down.

YELLS AND SCREAMS

Riders will often yell short commands or advice at you. These "barks" often seem rude and angry. Don't take yells and screams personally. Empathize with new riders—avoid yells and screams.

Pacelines and Echelons

DRAFTING IS EFFICIENT

Riding behind another rider takes less energy than "breaking the wind." At 25 mph about 20% less energy is required riding behind another rider when compared to riding on one's own.

LEARN THE RIGHT TECHNIQUES

Certain principles of riding in a group allow not only for increased efficiency of travel, but also for increased safety. Learn how to ride with a group of riders at moderate speed. You'll be able to better anticipate what happens when riding in fast packs.

PACELINES

Imagine five riders riding across the page:

Figure 16–1

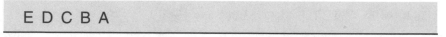

E D C B A

Rider A, finishing a turn at the front, swings to the left, slows down, and rider B takes the lead. Rider A drops in behind rider E.

Figure 16–2

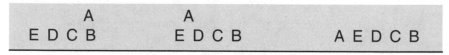

Shortly thereafter rider B does the same thing, and so on.

Figure 16–3

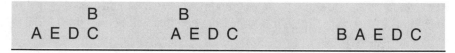

ECHELONS

If you are at all confused about pacelines, don't read this section.

Ride echelons only when you and your riding group are experienced in pacelines. Be careful to avoid pulling off the wrong way or you may find that overlapped wheels will result in a crash.

An echelon is staggered riding in a crosswind. Imagine the wind is coming from the bottom of the page. The riders traveling across the page will line up like this:

Figure 16–4

When A drops off, it will be by slowing down and drifting backwards. As B is overlapping his wheel, it will be by dropping off on the "windward" side:

Figure 16–5

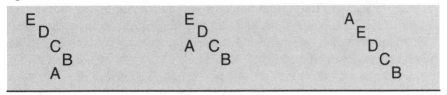

There is a limit to the number of riders that can ride an echelon, because road width is required to accommodate them.

Warming Up for Bicycling

Many riders and coaches believe in the value of a good warm-up. Although hard scientific evidence confirming the value of a warm-up may be lacking, warm-ups make good sense and are encouraged.

WHAT IS A WARM-UP?

For some it means stretching, then getting on the bike and slowly increasing effort in preparation for heavy exertion. Sometimes several hard jumps are included. In preparation for racing, several minutes (at least) of race speed effort are advised.

WHO WARMS UP? WHEN?

Many people seem to swear by the value of a good warm-up before training rides and races.

Ask any number of people about doing a time trial. Most will say that one of the most important things is a thorough, hard warm-up, so that you are ready to go hard from the first second. Same thing for criteriums. The shorter an event is, the more important it is to go hard from the start.

A stationary trainer may be a necessity for warming up if the race promoter is unable to provide a suitable area for this purpose.

WARM-UP SCIENCE

From a scientific point of view, the value of the warm-up is rationalized as a need to increase blood flow to the required muscle groups. Increased blood flow results in an increase in the local temperature of muscle cells which are working—making and using energy.

It is thought that heat might increase enzymatic activity in muscle groups/cells. Some think that heat may also serve to make muscle fibers less sticky (or viscous), allowing them to work more efficiently, and that fluids may increase in joints providing protection against injury.

Another reason given for a warm-up is to "loosen up" muscles, tendons, and ligaments so that there will be less chance of injury to these tissues.

Some studies have shown that sudden vigorous exercise places the heart at some risk for irregular rhythms and that warming up can help prevent this.

Neural patterns may be rehearsed, and training of neural patterns may make the activity easier to repeat.

Warm-up results in scientific studies are mixed. Confounding variables include motivation of the athlete, pain tolerance, performance techniques, and strategy.

A PERSONAL NOTE

It takes me many minutes of effort before my heart rate reaches its cruising time-trial speed. I can't blast off the line at the start of a race unless I've been riding for at least half an hour. When I get on my rollers, for the life of me, I can't maintain a cadence of 150 until I've been riding for at least 20 minutes.

Although little hard, scientific proof really exists about the value of warm-up, I think that it is important, and encourage you to try "hard" warm-ups. You may find that your performance improves.

Bumping

Beginning racers usually avoid all physical contact in their races. Race speeds and positioning in the more skilled categories often necessitate occasional contact. By practicing and becoming comfortable with physical contact, beginning racers acquire the skills needed for higher-level competition.

WHAT WE'RE TALKING ABOUT

Riding so close to another rider that you touch, bump into, and lean on each other.

Bumping is not a strategy for racing, but it is a part of any defensive bicycling skill program. By practicing this skill you will be less likely to panic if you are bumped in a race. By practicing, riders become more comfortable with proximity, or closeness, and become better pack riders.

Practice on a smooth grass field. Wear a helmet, long sleeves and pants, and gloves. As you acquire skill, practice on a velodrome or on the road.

Initially practice with a partner of similar height and weight. Choose a partner whose handlebars are about the same height as yours. The interlocking of handlebars is a cause of crashing; this risk is reduced when handlebars are the same height.

Ride side by side. Gently lean and bump shoulders and elbows. Look ahead, using only peripheral vision to see your partner.

As you become more comfortable, practice more intense bumps. Lean on your partner, don't merely touch. Your partner should be propping up your lean—you'd fall without your partner's counterpressure.

Switch sides and practice leaning and bumping the other side.

Play sandwich with two partners: Take turns riding in the middle, being bumped from both sides.

Touching Wheels

Almost all riders are afraid to touch wheels for fear of a crash. Wheel touching occasionally occurs in racing. By practicing wheel touching in a safe environment, skills can be acquired that increase the rider's chances of staying upright.

WHAT WE'RE TALKING ABOUT

Touching your front wheel against the rear wheel of another rider. The loss of steering control of the front wheel often causes a rider to crash. Overlapped wheels and rider panic in a race are a frequent cause of crashing.

But the overlapping and touching of wheels needn't spell disaster. There are techniques to disengage. By practicing this skill you will be less likely to panic if you touch wheels in a race. By practicing this skill, riders become more comfortable with the closeness encountered in the pack.

Practice on a smooth grass field. Wear a protective helmet, old cycling or street clothes with long sleeves and pants, and gloves.

Practice with one other rider.

One rider leads—rides straight, at a constant speed, listening to their partner, but not looking back. The lead rider is in minimal danger of crashing.

The rear rider matches the speed of the lead rider, and brings the front wheel up so it is just overlapping. The rear rider must not be as far advanced as the lead rider's hub. The rear rider positions the bike just an inch or two to the side of the lead rider's rear wheel, then taps or brushes the lead rider's rear wheel, then backs off.

The lead rider must continue to ride straight and steady—do not swerve, slow down, or speed up. The lead rider may be slowed slightly by the friction of the rear rider's front wheel.

In situations where there is more than just instantaneous contact, the rear rider must momentarily turn into the lead rider's rear wheel to set up the steering and lean of his own bicycle before disengaging.

It may sound backwards, but this counterintuitive technique is what allows skilled riders to avoid crashing. Try it and you'll see what I mean.

Practice touching from both the left and right sides.

Hill Technique—Ascending and Descending

Proper technique will get you up that hill faster and help you descend more quickly and with greater control and safety. Here are the salient features of climbing and descending.

STEADY LONG CLIMB

- Hands on the tops.
- Seat back.
- Push forward, not down.
- Concentrate on pulling up.
- Establish a breathing rhythm.
- Concentrate on your rhythm.
- Relax your arms.

OUT-OF-THE-SADDLE CLIMBING

- Hands on the brake hoods, a couple of fingers around the brake levers.
- As you push down with your left leg, pull up with the left arm/hand—most beginners do the opposite! As you pull with the left, relax your right grip and allow the bike to rock slightly to the right. Repeat on the right pedal stroke and you'll develop a comfortable climbing rhythm.
- Establish a breathing rhythm.
- Concentrate on your rhythm.

DESCENDING TECHNIQUE FOR CORNERS

- Dropping your torso lowers your center of gravity and speeds your descent. Raising your chest opens you to the wind and can be used as a mild wind break before the corner.
- Anticipate the speed for the corner and slow before the corner if necessary.
- Keep your hands in the drops, using a relaxed grip.
- Mildly unweight your rear end and move it slightly back on the saddle.
- When cornering, inside pedal up, outside pedal down.
- Straighten your outside leg and push down, putting weight on the outside pedal.
- Look beyond the turn.
- Ride outside-inside-outside: Approach the corner starting wide, cut to the apex, finish wide.
- Lean your bike more than your body by extending your inside arm, pressing down with your inside hand, straightening your body, leaning the bike.
- Pushing more with your inside hand to increase your lean will allow you to turn into the corner. Mildly unweighting your inside hand will allow you to turn out of the corner. This technique gives excellent adjustment and control to cornering.

Climbing

Hills are tough, but they are one of the best ways to make you stronger. By climbing efficiently with proper technique and within your abilities you'll get up faster and be happier. For many riders, good technique has made climbing their favorite form of cycling.

KNOW YOUR LIMITS

Know your strengths and weaknesses. How high can you go aerobically? For how long? Know your leg strength and how hard you can push. How long can you maintain a big gear?

RIDE STEADILY, STRAIGHT UP

The fastest way up is straight up. Weaving and winding your way up by traversing the width of the road may be necessary if you don't have a large enough cog, but it's slower that way.

If traffic is controlled, cutting corners shortens the distance you have to ride. Ride steadily. Avoid sprints (except as a training technique) on steady long climbs except near the end of the climb.

Knowing what you can do, and riding at a hard steady pace, is what gets you up fastest. If you work too hard you blow up, bog down, and end up miles behind.

RIDE AT THE FRONT IN GROUPS

It is better to be near the front of a pack on a climb and try to stay there, rather than trying to catch up from behind. There is no draft advantage to working from behind, and to catch up from behind you must work much harder than even the leaders of the hill climb.

If you position yourself at the front of a climbing pack, and you are going just a little slower than the strongest riders would if they were leading, most of the time stronger riders will not pass you and you will be able to stay with the pack on a hill a lot longer.

PLAN TO PUSH HARDER AT THE END

Good hill climbers shift to harder gears on the last half of the climb.

Unless you are the best climber, and leading the climb, climb in the lowest (easiest) gear you can, to keep up with the group. Closer to the top the pace increases. Shifts to harder gears are made, with the cadence remaining the same.

IN OR OUT OF THE SADDLE?

Some people say it's good to get out of the saddle when climbing; others say riding steadily in the saddle is best. It probably boils down to what you practice, and what works best for you.

Seated climbing is the most energy efficient. Climbing out of the saddle takes strength in the arms as well as the legs. It takes more energy, but you have more power. Try to direct your energy to those legs, and not waste energy on needless arm motion.

Standing while climbing relieves saddle soreness, and provides a change in position that can be helpful.

Again, climbing out of the saddle is less efficient, but gives you more power. If you want to attack, or you are in danger of being dropped and need that power, standing can help—just as when you need that power spurt in a sprint.

If you don't have the gears to spin up a hill, you may have no choice but to stand, even though it is not the most efficient way to climb.

CONSERVE IN A RACE

In-the-saddle climbing—spinning to stay with the group—is usually the best way to climb in a race. If you wish to string things out and are the strongest, or need extra power to keep up on a short section, a bigger gear or standing may help. Spinning seated saves the muscle power fibers for the last half of the hill, when the climb is tougher. It saves power fibers for the race's finishing sprint.

If you start at the front of a big group, and trickle slowly backwards, your effort up the climb may be less than the leaders, but you may still be able to maintain contact.

You have a certain amount of leg power available on every ride, like money in a bank account. You can only use up what's there.

HOW HARD CAN YOU PUSH?

When time trialing up a climb, or when you are the strongest rider, probably the fastest way up the climb is to climb with the biggest gear you can push.

Concentrate on pulling up as well as pushing. Try pushing forward with your leg, like a leg press, rather than down. Do you know your limits? Do you know what gear you can maintain? If your gear is too hard, and you bog down, you may lose gobs of time.

When climbing alone up a steady climb, or when climbing at your max, the most efficient cadence is probably between 50 and 70 rpm.

Cornering

Controlling the bicycle around a corner at speed requires special skill. In some races, the ability to corner quickly is the difference between winning and riding at the back of the pack.

As you speed around a corner, centrifugal force makes you want to fly out from the corner. In order to compensate, your center of gravity must lie inside the tire-road contact line. You have three basic choices, depending on your situation:

- You can angle both yourself and the bicycle. This is commonly called *leaning*.
- You can angle the bicycle more than your body. This is commonly called *countersteering*.
- You can angle your body more than the bicycle. This is commonly called *steering*.

Figure 16–6

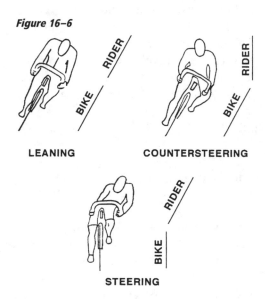

LEANING   COUNTERSTEERING

STEERING

For safety, when riding within a tight pack it's often important to corner the same way as others.

LEANING

Leaning through a corner is the most common method cyclists use. Both the bicycle and the rider are leaned into the corner. This method is suitable when the road is relatively wide, when you can see the roadway well after the corner, when you can choose your line ahead of time, and when the lean is brief—so that pedaling can resume after only a momentary, if any, pause.

COUNTERSTEERING

In *countersteering* you incline the bike relatively more than the body. You initiate countersteering by pressing down with the inside hand. This increases the lean of the bicycle into the turn. This method allows the most steering control and makes it easiest to affect a change in direction during the turn. It is suitable for when you cannot see the roadway around the turn, or for off-camber and decreasing-radius turns. The relatively large lean of the bike may prevent early pedaling. Countersteering is also especially suitable for descents where gravity, rather than pedaling, provides acceleration, and for changing and uncertain corners.

STEERING

Steering or turning the handlebar toward the turn and shifting your body weight to the inside of the bicycle allows the bicycle to remain relatively upright. This is helpful because you can continue to pedal around the corner. The relatively vertical wheels result in better bike control if sliding occurs. This is especially helpful in wet, oily, sandy, or gravelly conditions. For most riders this is an awkward and relatively slow way to corner. Repeated practice will improve speed. This is also the way one navigates in a pack—to either avoid potholes or pass slower riders—when learning is impractical.

HOW TO CORNER

For All Methods of Cornering

- Keep your hands in the drops, using a relaxed grip.
- Look beyond the turn to where you are going; do not look down at the ground.
- Drop your torso to lower your center of gravity.
- Anticipate the speed for the corner and slow before the corner if necessary.
- Ride outside-inside-outside: Approach the corner wide, cut to the apex, finish wide.
- Cutting too early is a common mistake. Cutting late allows you to see more road beyond the corner and to have more road on which to ride after making the turn.

For Leaning

- Employ the steps for all methods of cornering listed above.
- Mildly unweight your rear end and move it slightly back on the saddle.
- Have your inside pedal up, your outside pedal down.
- Straighten your outside leg and push down, putting weight on the outside pedal. In practicing this technique you can put all your weight on the outside pedal so that you are standing on it, and your rear end is off the saddle.
- The inside knee may be pointed toward the apex of the turn to help shift the center of gravity inside the tire line.

For Countersteering

- Employ the steps for all methods of cornering and leaning listed above.
- Lean your bike more than your body by extending your inside arm, pressing with your inside hand, keeping your body vertical and increasing the lean of the bike.

- Pushing more with your inside hand will allow you to turn more into the corner. Mildly unweighting your inside hand will allow you to turn out of the corner. The push is down to increase the lean of the bicycle, not forward to turn the wheel. This technique gives excellent adjustment and control to cornering.
- The inside hip may be rotated forward, and the inside knee may hug the top tube.

For Steering

- Employ the steps for all methods of cornering listed above.
- Keep the bicycle vertical.
- Shift your weight slightly forward and to the inside of the bicycle by shifting your hips and sitting more on the inside of your saddle.
- Straighten your outside arm, and push down and forward to turn, or steer, the bicycle.
- You may continue to pedal around the corner.

CORNERING DRILLS

- Choose a corner, a series of corners, or set up cones on grass or in a parking lot.
- Have a skilled rider draw the "ideal" line with chalk.
- Ride the corner alone.
- Ride following a skilled rider.
- Ride two abreast.
- Place a cone or chalk mark in the best line. Since sometimes other riders or hazards prevent you from riding the best line, learn how to take the next best natural line.

CHAPTER 17

Style

Anticipate, Don't React

Anticipation makes riding easier. Ever find yourself near the front of a group, feeling good and ready to make a move? Then, just as you got ready to jump, someone beat you to it. As they jumped, you had perfect timing and position to jump on their wheel. It was so easy! No gaps to close, no wind to fight, no extra effort required.

That kind of situation seems to develop infrequently for most riders. For others it seems to happen all the time.

Under such circumstances during a club training race one rider exclaimed, "For the first time in my life, I felt like I had everything going for me, and could win the race!"

Another rider I know wins crits all the time—riders always seem to jump just that split second before he does, and pull him off to victory, time and time again.

The crucial difference is anticipating moves—not having to close that 0.5- to 1-second gap due to late reaction, or, worse, too much of a delay, and then no possible reaction.

ACCORDION EFFECT

Driving your car, you get to a stoplight. If there are 10 cars ahead of you, it takes a long time after the light changes to green before you get to move. Each car is reacting not to the green light but to the movement of the car directly in front. The delay can take a half minute or longer. If the light changes back to red again in that half minute, you've lost several more minutes.

What if every driver started at precisely the same time. Sure, they'd be a lot closer to each other, and driving insanely, but they would all get through. You get the concept.

This is called the accordion effect. It is most pronounced at the back of the field in a tight criterium and spells disaster for most riders because it can cause them to get dropped out of the pack's draft, and hence out of the race. Each rider goes through the corner. Between each rider a little gap opens. Each little gap has to be closed.

It is easier to ride the front. But it really isn't necessarily that hard in the back—if you anticipate the cornering of the rider in front of you and have no gaps to close.

RIDERS ARE PREDICTABLE—ANTICIPATION CAN BE EASY

Try it. Anticipate the moves of your rivals. They have certain strengths and predictable moves. Packs are not mysterious. Anticipate the moves of the group. Packs have a predictable fluidity.

Be Aggressive, Not Passive

Aggressive riding is proactive riding. It means taking the initiative. It does not mean pushing, shoving, or dangerous riding.

AN EXAMPLE

Here's a situation to consider. Imagine a club racing exercise. A group of 10 riders divides into two teams of equal ability. Call them Team A and Team B. They start a practice race together. The object for each team is to get one of their team members to be the first to cross the finish line 10 miles down the road.

One of the members of Team A launches a rider off the front. Call him A1. Before anyone can react, he has a gap of 30 seconds. Team A naturally stops riding with any effort. Oops. Team B must do all the work and begin to chase down the A1 rider.

As soon as the group catches, or nearly catches, A2 and A3 from a break. They work together, and Team B has to continue to chase and to work. A2 and A3 also get caught, but now fresh A4 and A5 get away for good, and come in hand-in-hand to cross the finish line. First for Team A.

Both teams worked hard. All riders had to work. Team A had the advantage. It spent its time being aggressive, and its moves counted. Team B was passive. They had to work to chase. There's just as much work in chasing, but less glory.

Team B was always behind Team A, always playing catch-up. The winner is the team whose rider crossed the line first, not the team that chased the most. Who worked the most is irrelevant.

AGGRESSIVE RIDING IS EASIER

Ever felt you were one of the strongest riders on a ride? Felt like making the others hurt? Tried jumping up little rises and attacks off the front? Everyone else had to react, or be left behind. If your efforts were relatively short, and the group behind did not work well together, they had to work just as hard as you. Only they were behind, and you were ahead.

What about the opposite situation in a race? Felt intimidated by out-of-town racers? Did you let them jump and dictate the race? Did you let them control things, forcing you to react? Always feeling a little behind?

Are you a good time trialist, good in pursuit, but a lousy sprinter? What about that crit where the pace slows down a lap or so before the finish, where all the sprinters jockey for position? And what are you doing—the same thing, trying to get on a good wheel? Only you are not a sprinter. Oops. You are in trouble. You don't have a chance in the sprint! You are being too passive.

TRY AGGRESSIVE RIDING

Be aggressive. Maybe it won't work every race, maybe not even 25% of the races. But if you are a strong time trialist and lousy sprinter, try jumping with a lap or two to go. So what if you end up with egg on your face? You didn't have a chance in that sprint, no matter what you told your friends. Maybe you can win a crit!

Energy Conservation

Every expenditure of energy in a race should have a purpose. Ideally, no energy will be wasted. Smart riding means that when you work you have a tactical reason for doing so.

SAVE ENERGY

It's good for the planet, and it's good for you as a bike racer. I am not suggesting that you train this way. Racing is different. When you don't need to use energy, don't. Remember: Every expenditure of energy should have a purpose.

WASTING ENERGY

A new racer was feeling great. The pack was traveling 26 miles per hour and she felt strong. She went off the front halfway through the race, and was caught two short laps later.

"What were you thinking?" I asked.

"Well, I was feeling real good. I felt I had a lot of energy. I felt I could go a lot faster. I just took off."

"How fast was the pack going?" I asked.

"26 miles per hour," she answered.

"How much time was left in the race?"

"About 15 minutes."

"How fast can you time-trial?"

"About 25 miles per hour."

"So where were you going?" I asked.

"I see," she said.

HOW TO SAVE ENERGY

- Pulling the entire pack into a headwind might seem macho, but there are no prizes for the rider who pulls the most.
- If a climb is coming up, pulling the pack to the base of it is likely to make the hill a whole lot harder for you. Jumping the pack, getting a good gap, and then climbing the hill at a more moderate pace is a different tactic that has occasional merit.
- Riding behind small riders doesn't provide the same draft as sheltering in the wake of thunder-thighed giants.
- All riders are fresh at the start of the race. After the race is half over, some have had mechanical problems, some are spent, and most are tired. In the first half of the race, many people have the ability to stay with your efforts. In the last half, fewer can respond. Your efforts will make more of a difference. If you are definitely one of the strongest, you may want to toughen the race from the start. But most early attacks are pointless, except for the desperate.

CRITERIUM ENERGY CONSERVATION

- Position yourself properly. There's a lot of fighting for position at the immediate front of a pack. Often this takes mental as well as physical energy. Things may be a lot smoother 10 or 20 riders back.
- Crits with long straights and few technical corners can be ridden efficiently at the back. But you run the risk of a winning break disappearing up the road. Shorten the straights and make those corners more often than every tenth of a kilometer, however, and the accordion effect will whip you off the back. Stay at the front.
- Decelerate, if necessary, before corners. Begin accelerating again before or during the corner. You will then have the momentum to continue accelerating after the corner.
- Learn to recognize potentially successful breakaways. Don't waste your energy in those doomed to failure.

CLIMBING ENERGY CONSERVATION

- Try to start the climb at the front of the pack.
- If there is no danger of a break getting away, sliding to the back of the pack can save a lot of energy. The more riders in the pack, the more energy you can save.

BREAKAWAY ENERGY CONSERVATION

- Paceline work in a break is full of tactics. Don't get behind the strongest rider. Choose the slowest rider who won't get dropped.

- Don't be right in front of the strongest rider, getting back on to the line may be difficult.
- Don't point yourself out by taking charge—everyone will notice you and your efforts.
- You can be modest and feign some weakness. Snappy accelerations make you a marked rider.

WHEN TO USE ENERGY

- When it matters. When it counts.
- When it allows you to break away.
- When it forces the others to work too, softening them up.
- When you can capitalize on the weaknesses of your opponents.
- When it helps your teammates.
- When you have the element of surprise, the right timing.
- When you can carry it through.
- When you have no choice if you want to preserve your chances.

CHAPTER 18

Tactics

Attacking

An attack is a hard effort meant to leave other riders behind. It is just the opposite of riding steadily. It is just the opposite of "working together with a group." It is working separately to achieve some goal.

The goal may be to get away solo. It may be to separate and weaken the field, it may be to race out for a prime, it may be to separate from the peloton and join the break. It may be to encourage another rider to chase for the purpose of allowing a counterattack by a teammate. Or, the goal may simply be to test other riders and see who responds.

An attack is like a sprint, in the sense that it requires a sudden burst of energy. Gradual increases in effort are not attacks—that's called pulling. A gradual increase in effort that sheds other riders is not an attack, it's called superior strength and dropping other riders. Attacking involves a sharp increase in speed.

TIMING

As in gymnastics, it's not only strength, it's how you use that strength that's important. Timing is often everything in an attack. Here are some situations which may present an opportunity for an attack:

- Near the top of a climb.
- When another rider or group is caught.
- After a prime or intermediate points sprint.
- When corners or twists in the road allow an escape to be "out of sight, out of mind."
- On the lee side of the wind when the strongest or threat rider is trapped by the rest of the paceline.
- When a teammate pulls off the paceline or is in front of the paceline, blocking others.
- When a crash or other disruption in the pack occurs.
- At the feed zone.*
- When a car or truck passes on a non-closed road, which gains you a temporary draft.*
- Just before a corner, chopping the corner.*

PREDICTABLE ATTACKS

Some of the above situations are very predictable—riders often attack when using their strength means that if others are going to respond to the attack they must use up energy as well. For example, climbers attack on hills or strong time trialists attack and form echelons in strong crosswinds.

Riders also predictably attack when others have worked hard and they haven't, as in a counterattack—after an attack has been caught or after a prime in a criterium.

Even though predictable, such attacks may be effective because they occur when others are tired and must match the effort of the attack to respond. If riders are not strong, they will fail to neutralize the attack.

SURPRISE ATTACKS

Attack at an unexpected time when others think it's not likely to work.

Consider this scenario: There are 200 yards to the top of a climb, then 1 mile straight downhill into the wind, a couple of corners, and finally 3 flat miles to the finish.

The race might be for the corners, but no one is going to attack downhill into the wind. *Everyone* knows that a pack is faster than an individual going downhill, especially into the wind.

* Considered by some to be unsporting.

Roll away on the last part of the climb, and pedal smoothly, in an apparently non-attacking way, downhill. The pack may not react because a single rider can't get very far alone downhill into the wind.

Can they not? Sure—if the rider works hard (albeit smoothly and not necessarily noticeably) and the pack is letting everyone else go into the wind first. Really punch around the corners and get out of sight. Some riders in the pack might have trouble believing there is anyone up the road!

Other Surprisingly Effective Times to Attack

- *Into a tailwind*. Everyone feels great in a tailwind. Escapes are often difficult. On the other hand, when a super time trialist goes, it forces everyone to work, and the riders drop one by one, preventing them from working again together. In a crit, attacking into the tailwind side can give you extra time: Normally a crit pack does not get organized into a headwind—they normally organize on the tailwind side. Timed right, an attack into a tailwind may give a bigger gap because the initial disorganization that accompanies many attacks means the pack won't organize for a full lap—the next tailwind section. You may have an extra half lap in which to work.
- *Into a headwind*. Who would dare? On the other hand, who wants to chase you, using their energy to pull the rest of the pack along? Another chance for a time trialist to go.
- *Before the climb*. Can give you extra time to get up the climb. The climbers may save it for the climb. But you may have such a gap as to be enough ahead to get to the top before them. This works best into a little bit of headwind and in small fields. With large fields, the momentum of the pack is so large that you are likely to be swallowed up and waste your energy.
- *Just after you've been caught*—if you've tempered your efforts before being caught. Who would expect it?

SNEAK ATTACKS

A strong attack sometimes discourages others and gains an immediate gap. But a strong attack is perceived as a real threat—which of course it may be.

An attack is often defined as a hard effort meant to leave behind or weaken others. Some coaches advise never to attack half-heartedly—attacks should be sharp, solid actions.

I disagree. There are times when it's best to camouflage one's attack—to make an effort to separate yourself from others, but not so obvious an effort as to be perceived as a threat.

After all, it takes considerable strength to move away from the field, especially when they are watching you.

Sometimes it is possible to separate oneself without worrying others. This is a key point in many successful moves: Other riders feel they could match your efforts, but as they don't feel threatened, they see no need to do so. Here are some examples:

- *Roll off the front.* A sharp increase in speed is noticed. But if you slowly increase the tempo, it's possible the others will stay at their own speed, and not realize that you are creating a gap. Since your effort is not perceived as a threat, you may just roll away. Strong time trialists can catch the pack napping, and gain considerable distance before riders realize it: "Hey, he's pretty far out there, and we're not gaining on him—he's rolled away."
- *Lull your opponents into a false sense of security* by making apparently unsuccessful false attacks. If your repeated efforts get you nowhere, people may stop noticing them. Then you can really make the effort that counts, and riders will figure the same low-level response will get you back—which, for your serious effort, will not.
- *Make your offensive move appear defensive.* Cover a break or an attack which makes your move appear defensive, when it's really an attack or offense of your own.

From what I saw on TV of the women's 1996 Olympic road race, one could easily imagine this scenario: The whole pack is watching Jeannie Longo, worried about an attack and ready to cover her. An Italian is off the front. She gets reeled in, and another Italian attacks. Jeannie Longo jumps to cover the attack. Now she's on the defensive, covering someone else's attack. . . . Oh no! It's not defensive. Now Jeannie's got a gap, working with the Italian, and turning an apparent defensive move into an offensive one.

POSITION FOR ATTACKING

It's easier to attack from the back of a small group or about a third of the way back in a larger group. If you attack from the front, everyone can see what you are doing and you won't have the element of surprise to help you open a gap.

If you attack from behind a small group, it is even easier if you let a small gap open, and attack into the gap, and then around the group. Then you can accelerate into the draft of the group and come around with even greater speed, allowing you to open a lead more quickly and with less effort.

Gapping

Most riders understand how attacking and working hard is a tactic that uses *one's own* energy to gain an advantage. Relatively few appreciate how powerful a tactic gapping riders can be—forcing others to work and using *their* energy to gain an advantage.

Gapping is letting some space open between you and the rider in front of you. Timed right, it can accomplish minor miracles.

INDIVIDUAL RIDER GAPS TO REARRANGE A BREAK OR LAUNCH AN ATTACK

Gapping can be used as a tactic without a team. With a teammate, it can be devastating to an opponent of superior ability. Let's consider a few examples, first without teammates:

Figure 18–1

Riders X, Y, and A are all about equal in strength and speed. Then, 300 meters from the finish line, riders X, Y, and A get ready to sprint. Rider A lets a gap open on rider Y.

Figure 18–2

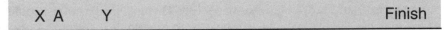

This can be useful for two reasons. First, in a race situation, most X's would get antsy, and work to catch Y, towing A along. Rider X would be required to work harder than A to catch Y. Both X and Y would break the wind. Rider A could work the least, and launch a winning sprint 150 meters from the line.

Second, if the gap were not too large, rider A might accelerate into Y's draft at the critical moment to whip around Y with greater speed than he might otherwise accomplish. With enough speed and timing, he might prevent X from coming around him to win.

GAPPING WITH A TEAMMATE

A and B ride a tandem. C works with the tandem. A and B have an advantage on the tandem, with good high-end speed and endurance. Unfortunately, they aren't the greatest sprinters.

When X rides, A and B need help to get away. Once away, they can stay away, but how to get X off their draft? C makes it easy—C gaps A and B at just the right moment!

Figure 18–3

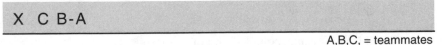

A,B,C, = teammates

Just as A and B accelerate, C appears to be increasing his speed, but then fizzles:

Figure 18–4

X C	B-A

X is a far better sprinter than A, B, or C, but that gap, made at just the right moment with the help of C, gives the tandem just enough distance to allow it to leave behind even a most determined X.

Timing is everything. C has to leave a gap just precisely when A and B work their hardest to jump away. This takes practice.

GAP FORCES OTHERS TO WORK HARDER OR HELPS A TEAMMATE

Gapping helps A win the Tour of Studs. There are seven riders off the front of the field. A has both B and C to help. He's as strong as they come, but has no sprint.

Figure 18–5

W X C Y Z B A

A,B,C, = teammates

If everyone stays on A's wheel and does nothing, A will tow the group. Riders will come around a tired A at the sprint finish. Everyone is working near max. Rider A does not have enough speed to attack successfully away from the group. What to do? Open a gap!

Figure 18–6

W X C Y Z B   A

A is now out front, and it takes an anaerobic effort for Z to come around B and close the gap.

Figure 18–7

W X C Y B Z A

Rider A maintains his steady, relentless pace. Z is a little pooped after his effort, and hasn't the willpower to resist B's intrusion into his place. Pooped, Z goes to the back of the pack.

Figure 18–8

```
Z W X C Y B A
```

B does the same thing to Y. Another gap opens:

Figure 18–9

```
Z W X C Y B     A
```

Now Y is forced to come around, go anaerobic, and tow up to A.

This gets repeated several more times with Y and Z. Remember everyone is working close to their anaerobic threshold. Y and Z have had to exceed theirs several times.

W and X could care less about chasing down A—they let Z in ahead of them the next time B forces him off A's wheel. Once again Y is on B's wheel. Once again B gaps, and A is off.

Figure 18–10

```
        W X Z C Y B          A
```

Again Y is forced to chase. This time he's a little too tired from his previous anaerobic efforts. He pulls part of the way up to A, then pulls off, looking for help to chase down A.

Figure 18–11

```
                    B Y
                    W X Z C     A
```

Now C, A's other teammate, is in the front of the pack. But he doesn't pull. He just sits there, not working.

Z is cooked, Y is cooked, W and X aren't really in the game, and A is away. He wins, solo.

PACK DYNAMICS

Normally in a race you can count on a couple of riders to try to counter an attack (Y and Z) or catch your teammates, and at least an equal number (W and X) of "neutral riders"—the sheep on automatic drafting pilot, who would just as soon sit in, save it for the sprint, survive, whatever. It may not take more than a couple of riders to control the pack.

Blocking

Blocking is a tactic used to slow down a group of riders. It is a very important tactic when for any of several different reasons it becomes advantageous to slow down the group.

CONSIDER THESE POSSIBILITIES

1. The team has a very strong rider who is trying to get away. She's an excellent time trialist, with excellent endurance. Suppose the team wants her to win. We get her off the front and then try to slow everybody else down.
2. We want to try and set up one of our sprinters. But this sprinter does not have very good high-end endurance, and if the pace stays too high for too long, she'll burn up. Blockers serve to interfere with the smooth functioning of the group and slow the pace to allow our sprinter to sit in and win at the end.

TYPES OF BLOCKING

There are many methods of blocking. Keep in mind that should the other riders of the group be aware of your actions, or other racers wish the group to go faster, you may not be popular. It is sometimes necessary to put up with some abuse when you are a blocker, or be crafty so others don't realize what's happening. In any situation, blocking should never be performed erratically or in an unsafe manner.

Criterium Blocking

Get to the corners first. Take outside to inside lines, slow down. The pack accordions shut instead of open.

Mass Team Blocking

Everyone on your team to the front. Go slow. This works best on narrow roads.

Passive Blocking

Take your pull when you come to the front of the pack, but don't pull off. Slow down little by little, so that the pack's speed falls. If you slow down too much, too quickly, other riders will be wise to you and pass you when you come to the front of the pack, making your blocking efforts less effective.

Active Blocking

Stay about second or third in the pack. Jump on any wheel as it comes by. Refuse to work, refuse to pull. Mess up the rhythm of the group. As soon as another rider comes by to pull and increase the speed of the pack, jump on the new lead rider's wheel. When he pulls off, pull off with him, or beside him—wreck the speed of the group.

This is a favorite method. You get an excellent workout at the same time. In a criterium you get about three or four jumps in every single mile.

But it is not the way to make friends in the pack. You have to be careful, for other riders may try to hook you, elbow you, and abuse you verbally or otherwise.

Still, taken in the right spirit, it's great training, and most riders, when they do understand what you are doing—even if they don't like it—don't take it personally.

"Fred" Method

I don't recommend this method—but since some riders use it, it is helpful to be aware of it. If you choose this method, be sure you are riding safely.

Act like a total clod. It helps to wear tube socks. Pretend you don't know how to ride a bike straight. Perhaps weave a little. Riders may not want to ride near you.

I've known a rider or two to actually win this way, keeping other riders from passing him, until he was ready and able to sprint for the finish.

Blocking by Talking

This happens all the time. Engage the leaders in conversation about this or that. Ask questions. Some riders may be too polite or unfocused about the race, slow down, actually reply, and waste energy.

Distraction Talking

Get near the front of the group, but not at the front. Start talking about the weather, wildflowers, or pets. Open up a political, religious, or other controversial discussion. Talk about crime, abortion, or health care. You may get other riders to forget about racing or chasing or otherwise distract them.

Sitting-on Blocking

Sit in the back of the chase group. Do absolutely no work. The others may get so frustrated and mad, worrying about you not working, that you may discourage their progress.

Teamwork

Teamwork means many different things. It means training with friends, it means traveling to races with friends, it means working toward a common goal. What I am concerned with here is how to work effectively as a team, toward a common goal, in a race.

TEAMWORK IS SELFLESS RIDING

Teamwork means that although you care about your personal performance, you are willing to help your teammates. This may mean riding harder or more easily than you would without them being present. The heart of teamwork is realizing that together we are much stronger than we are individually.

An Example

Consider this setup: Two strong teammates are in a break with an extremely strong opponent. Call the teammates T1 and T2. Call the opponent E for the enemy. Back in the pack are several other teammates, T3, T4, and T5.

Up in the break, T1, T2, and E are working together, and in the chasing peloton T3, T4, and T5 are sitting in, not doing any work, and so making the other riders work harder to catch the break.

TEAM FINISH

Up at the front, T1 jumps off by herself just as E finishes a strong pull. T2 has positioned herself behind E. T1 goes away to win solo.

Or maybe not. Maybe E chases T1 down, and just as T1 is caught, T2 accelerates and goes off to win solo.

Or no, E chases again, T1 tucks in on her wheel, and just as T2 is caught, T1 goes again, this time for good, E being finally too tired to chase.

Done right, it is almost a certainty that T1 or T2 will win. Left to a field sprint—well, E is a national-caliber sprinter. The team would prefer not to take the chance of a sprint finish, and doesn't need to!

COUNTERTACTICS?

If E attacked earlier, solo, it wouldn't have done her any good, because T1 and T2 are stronger together than she is alone. If after T1 originally attacked, E then chased hard, momentarily dropping T2, that wouldn't matter a great deal, either—T1 could just sit on E's wheel, E would probably slow down, and T1 and E would be left waiting for T2 to catch. Then it's two on one again!

If the chase group worked extremely hard to catch while these shenanigans were going on, it might not be so bad, either. Fresh T3, T4, or T5 could attack separately or together and work to either win or force another chase.

TEAMWORK SECRET

The secret is working together. T1, T2, T3, T4, and T5 not minding—rather, enjoying—their teammate's success! Riders feel good when their teammates do well.

SELFLESS RIDING IS SELFISH RIDING TOO

By helping their teammates, riders also improve their own chances.

Take the above example with T1, T2, and E. Suppose they were by far the three strongest in the race, and about equal. Independently, their chances of winning might be said to be 1 in 3.

With teamwork, T1 and T2 destroy E's chances. Now T1 and T2 have improved their odds to 1 in 2.

BASIC TEAMWORK

Beginning team racers often want to help, but don't know exactly how. Keep it simple. On the most basic level, it boils down to the following:

Chase Opponents

If some other team has a break with their riders in it, and you don't have a teammate in the break, or your teammate is disadvantaged in the break, and if the pack is not working to chase down the break, work to chase down the break.

Don't Chase Teammates

If a teammate is off the front, or a preponderance of team members are in a break, sit in and do as little work as possible.

TEAMWORK WITHOUT TEAMMATES

You may race without teammates. But it's possible to play the peloton in such a way as to effectively have a dozen or more teammates. Here's how to do it!

If you find yourself without teammates and adopt a passive role, the lack of teammate support may hurt your chances.

If you are a relatively strong rider, and in the hunt for a place or win, it's possible to work the field and have many others help you.

Basic Principles

- Every expenditure of energy should have a purpose.
- Letting the pack work against you lessens your chances for success.
- Letting the pack work for you improves your chances.
- The more riders you can get to work hard while you rest the better your chances when you play your cards.

An Example

I traveled out of town to a regional championship. The race was a rolling 2-mile circuit, 20 laps. I knew I probably was one of the strongest. I wasn't sure who the other players were.

Each lap, I moved to the front as we rolled toward the most significant climb. As we came to the corner that began the start of the climb, I let a gap open on three or four riders.

These riders would normally get up the climb first. I slip-slided, climbing a little slower than everyone else, conserving energy. The pack was large enough that on the rolling downhill the leaders could be caught without too much effort. Usually, I'd make it down the hill at the front again, and slow the chase just a little through the corners.

Each lap I let three riders work hard, escape, and work together to try and get away. Each lap four or five other riders worked to chase them down. Each lap a few more riders blew off the back. After about 15 laps, one of the riders, annoyed at those gaps, yelled, "What the hell are you doing!"

By the time the closing laps came around, I had done lots of tactical work, but hardly any anaerobic efforts. The strong riders had worked quite hard. I had let my "teammates" off the front repeatedly. I had let my other "teammates" chase them down. They had all helped me save my energy.

When it came down to the end, I had the most energy left!

After the race the rider who had yelled at me came up and said, "You were riding as if you were protecting your teammates off the front. You let them go, you gapped them off. You even did some blocking in the chases. But they weren't really your teammates!"

I told him that in several years of racing he was the first rider to have figured out this strategy and discussed it with me. It was as if a light went on, and he smiled and said, "Next time you're racing here, count on me—you'll really have a teammate!"

Wheelsuckers

There is a great deal of admiration for the strongest one in the group, the one who can time-trial faster than anyone else. There's glory in being able to climb and climb, dropping your rivals one by one. Some folks castigate the wheel-sucker, believing that racer to be the basest form of lowlife on the planet—it's an unfair rap!

YELLING IN THE PELOTON

Ever notice how much yelling and screaming go on in a pack? When yells are directed at novices, it's usually because they are riding dangerously with respect to codes of pack safety. When shouting to teammates, it's usually a request for help. When yelling at rivals, it is usually not because anyone is doing anything wrong. It's because someone is doing something different than the yeller wants.

"People yell at me in a race when I don't do enough to help them win!" said Nelson Cronyn, one of the country's best time trialists.

CLIMBERS

Ever notice how climbers always want the group to ride steadily on the flats? "Hey, keep it smooth," they shout. It's not really that the ride should neces-sarily be smooth, it's that they, the climbers, want the group to stay intact until the hills, when they can say, "See ya!"

TIME TRIALISTS

Notice how the time trialists say to the climbers, "Keep it together on the hills. When we get to the flats, we can really work together." Of course, after the climb they can show off, towing the group at warp speed, and gloating at their strength.

One of the legends of our club was a time trialist extraordinaire, and a good climber to boot. He'd ride away from fields and never be seen again. If there was a sprint finish he was dead meat. Naturally enough he hated wheelsuckers and swore at them every chance he got.

PACK FODDER

The majority of riders are neither great climbers nor great time trialists. They ride club rides, rolling road races, and crits. As long as they have the basic fitness to be with the pack, they can be "boxed out," have a "bad day," or who knows what in the final few laps—but hey, they were there!

SPRINTERS

Then there is that ability to sprint. To go warp speed for 200 to 1,000 meters and win races. "Fast finishers," they call 'em. Maybe not a great climber, maybe not a good time trialist. There is more to winning sprints than speed. A crucial asset of a winning sprinter is positioning—that is, sucking on the right wheels until the last possible moment.

Climbers are great, and they dislike wheelsuckers who beat 'em in the sprint. Time trialists are strong, and they dislike wheelsuckers who come around 'em at will (though ever so briefly). Pack riders dislike wheelsuckers because they show 'em up at the end of races.

WHEELSUCKERS ARE POSITION SPECIALISTS

The wheelsucker gets a bad rap, but what a talent! A talent different from time trialing, different from hill climbing, but talent!

SUCCESSFUL WHEELSUCKING EXAMPLES

I remember a Wednesday coast ride with a bunch of exceptionally strong local racers. I sat in all the way and beat them all in the sprint. "My mother could have won that sprint with all your wheelsucking," yelled one of them. "Hey," I said under my breath, "if you've got a mother with genes like that, what are you yelling about!"

And then there was a World Week Handicap Race in Austria, where I wheelsucked behind a national champion all the way to the front of the race and then beat him in the sprint. Boy, was he sore! But hey, he was motoring and never pulled over for me to lead, so I just tagged along for the ride. What did he expect me to do? Say "Thanks," and then let him win?

THE BIG NAMES WHEELSUCK TOO

Greg LeMond has won the World Championships. Does he do anything the first 80% of the race? Of course not. Nada. He lets the race unfold, he's patient, and when everyone is suitably pooped, he goes to the front.

Andy Hampsten rode a magnificent finish to win Alp d'Huez back in the 1992 Tour de France—a climber's lifelong dream. What did he say? "I did as little work as possible on the days leading up, letting myself rest as much as possible to give everything to this stage." That is to say, he wheelsucked ad nauseam until his moment of glory.

Look at old footage of Davis Phinney and Ron Kiefel. Phinney, the cash register, winning more primes and finishes than any other racer. Does he go out alone time trialing with 20 laps to go? Does he win KOM points? Nyet. He lets his teammates guard for breaks, works in breaks when needed, but sucks on Kiefel's wheel until the time is right to make his move.

THE BEST WHEELSUCKERS ARE NOT NOTICED

Remember only the engine, that one person at the front, is working. Every one else is sucking.

A local club racer tears up the crit circuit, and few notice he hardly ever pulls when not needed. He's a wheelsucker par excellence. Others are often noticed wheelsucking and get yelled at. Try and wheelsuck without notoriety!

DON'T TAKE WHEELSUCKERS PERSONALLY

Yelling at wheelsuckers may be a valid tactic, and occasionally it works. Don't let them get to you, though, and don't take it personally.

Truthfully, a wheelsucker should be admired. Wheelsucking is a real talent, and one that can be as valuable as time trialing or climbing. A good wheelsucker is an invaluable teammate in almost any race.

WHEELSUCKERS, TAKE CARE

If you are a wheelsucker, be aware that others may be annoyed by you. Wheelsuckers have a habit of being ridden into the gutter, or worse. Dangerous riding is always unacceptable, but wheelsuckers frustrate many riders into doing unacceptable things.

GETTING RID OF A WHEELSUCKER SAFELY

When you are a climber or a time trialist, how do you get rid of a wheelsucker?

- Out-climb 'em.
- Jump 'em and out-time-trial 'em.
- Work with others, let gaps open, and trap them on the wrong end of those gaps.

There is only one thing worse than a pure wheelsucker: That's a wheelsucker who can climb and time-trial too!

Successful Breakaways

Many riders wonder why the breakaways they are in never seem to succeed, whereas the ones they don't make frequently work. It's not really such a mystery. Successful breakaways are predictable.

WHAT WE'RE TALKING ABOUT

A small group of riders manages to escape off the front of the criterium you are riding, and stay away. Earlier you were in two separate breakaways, neither of which worked. Why is it just now, when you are resting, that this break eludes you?

There are many elements that factor into winning breakaways. Once you understand these elements, winning breakaways are much more predictable.

FREQUENT FLYERS

The riders in successful breakaways include the stronger riders. For a break to work, it must travel faster than the pack. If the strong riders are in the pack, and reasonably alert, they will probably band together to chase down breaks of weak riders.

Successful break riders aren't only lucky. They are persistent. Repeated breakaway attempts improve the odds.

CATEGORIES PREDICT BREAKAWAYS

In Categories 4 and 5 the very strong riders may ride off the front. That's not really a breakaway. It's the disappearance of the chaff. The Cat 3's are fairly uniform in strength, having risen up from the Cat 4's, but are not yet strong enough for the 1,2's. Relatively few breaks occur in this category.

The 1,2's have no place to go. To a Cat 5, all 1,2's are strong, but there are big differences in ability. Same thing in age-graded racing. Local masters 40+ races can have a couple of Cat 1's mixed in with some Cat 5's. This is where successful breakaways most often occur.

RIGHT TEAMS

Successful breakaways have the right combination of teams represented. Some teams definitely have a few good players. The successful break needs representatives from a few of the good teams, or else the good riders left behind will work together to destroy the breakaway's chances.

Alternatively, a missing team might send a rider up to bridge or join the break. Now the chances for the break's success have increased. Having the right combination of teams represented does not just apply to the breakaway group; it also means that teammates back in the pack will help in blocking and impeding the progress of the chasing pack.

THE COURSE MATTERS

Some courses lend themselves to breaks. A break can usually take a corner faster than the pack so courses with lots of corners help breaks. Road courses that are rolling or twisty are also good for breaks since it lets them get out of sight and out of mind. Success here is more likely than on a course with long straights and a lot of road visible ahead.

BREAK MEMBERS MUST WORK

Breakaway companions must begin to work immediately. A gap of at least 15 seconds is a must in crits. A single strong rider from the pack can close a 15-second gap. It's hard for teammates to block a gap that small. Larger gaps require the concerted effort of several pack members and are much harder to close.

The breakaway members must share the desire to work. One local national champion, a very strong rider, often escapes with a breakaway. Although he prefers solo escapes, it is common to see him work hard with a break. Some of the breaks he's in don't work and fall apart. Predictably, if a sprinter has made the break with him, our national champion is unwilling to work. He's wary of being outsprinted so he'll let the break be reabsorbed, and try for a different combination of riders later.

Some strong teams have certain predictable strategies. One very strong local team only works in breaks in the last half of a race. If you escape with a few of their riders early on, their members will just sit in. You've wasted your energy.

TIMING HELPS

Breaks may arise at the start of a race, but most successful breaks form with a third or less of the race to go. At the start everyone is present, and all are fresh. After half the race has passed, some riders have had mechanicals, and some may have crashed. In the last half, riders without endurance who might have chased down breaks in the first half are toast, and don't have the desire to respond to surges and breaks.

Successful breaks often work when the pack is lethargic or wary. After a couple of crit laps with contested primes, the pack is relatively tired. Breaks have more chance of succeeding now that everyone is not fresh.

Working Your Breakaway

There is more to being in a breakaway than working hard. *How* you work governs the breakaways and your chances for success.

WILL THE BREAK WORK?

The first question to consider before expending your energy is: Why waste your energy if the break's chances are doomed?

ESTABLISH AN EARLY GAP

You need a gap of at least 15 seconds in a standard criterium. Do it quickly—15 seconds is the gap that individual strong riders can close either by pulling or by bridging.

WORK EFFICIENTLY AS A GROUP

A successful breakaway is like a team time trial. Ride smoothly without surges. Pull off after the corner, not before—it is more efficient for the group. If you must pull off before the corner, do so to the outside, not the inside.

Larger riders break the wind more efficiently for the group as a whole than do smaller riders. Let larger riders pull into the wind, and smaller riders pull without wind, into tailwinds or uphill.

SECURE THE BREAK

After the break is secured, you can afford to consider other possibilities. The break is considered secured when a gap of sufficient distance has been established so that individuals within the break could continue to gap the pack if working alone. Only after the break is secured should you consider coy behavior.

IS THERE A DRIVING FORCE?

The driving force is not necessarily the strongest rider. Breakaways often need a conductor to make sure everyone is working, or to make sure that rival teams don't try to outmaneuver each other to the detriment of the break. If someone has taken that role, you can disappear in the break and hide some strength.

HOW HARD MUST YOU WORK?

If you are a weaker rider, be realistic—you must ride efficiently and conserve energy. If you are a stronger rider, you must decide whether to use your energy to give the break a maximum gap, attack the break, or ride efficiently for later moves. Stronger riders have the option of nursing weaker riders along, protecting them and the break.

ENERGY CONSERVATION

There are ways to take your pulls and yet work less than your partners. This is important if you are a weaker rider in the break.

Positioning yourself behind the strongest rider may be unwise. The strongest rider may pull the hardest and longest. When it is your turn to pull, you may already be tired. Positioning yourself behind the weakest rider who won't get dropped is an energy-conserving move. The rider with the broadest hips usually provides the best draft. Better drafts mean less work for you.

Keeping pace and pulling into the wind is very demanding. In a criterium, breaks often develop a rhythm and some riders seem to always pull on the headwind leg. It need not be you.

If the course has a hill, don't pull too hard in the section leading to the climb. You may need all your energy to keep up.

Criterium Solo Breakaway

Winning a race by a solo breakaway is a high point for almost any racer. Here's how to do it!

REQUIREMENTS

Winning a criterium race by a solo breakaway has several requirements:

Fitness

Let's face it—if you are struggling at the back of the crit, nearly max'd out, today is probably not going to be your day to go off the front.

While sheltered in the pack, you need to be about 20 beats below your anaerobic threshold in order to be able to travel at the pack's pace on your own.

It may seem easy in the pack's shelter, but check you computer. If the pack's going at 27 mph and you can't time-trial faster than that, where do you think you are going?

Timing

There are almost no riders who can make their escape at will. Riders who time-trial many miles an hour slower than you can suck on your wheel, benefiting from your slipstream, using 30% or so less energy. You don't want that. You don't want to be pulling. There's no prize for the rider who pulls the most. You want a clean break before you start time trialing off the front.

If you really are one of the strongest—one who is able to make a solo break stick—look for a time when you've been sheltered but the pack as a whole has been working pretty hard. A good example of this situation is when the pack has just finished chasing down an earlier break. Those weaker than you should be beyond their threshold, and not able to respond.

Primes provide opportunities. If the pack thinks you are going for a prime, you may escape. If you keep going, no one may be on your wheel, and when they realize you are not going to let up, it may be too late for them to catch you.

Or if riders are going for a prime, you can counter just after the prime, as they sit up.

A teammate can help. Your teammate attacks, and is chased. The moment he is caught, counter.

You can arrange it all yourself. Let a few strong riders go—say, by opening a gap rounding a corner. Those few in front may realize they have a little gap and be willing to work. A few strong riders left in the pack may work to catch up. Counterattack as the break gets caught. Or bridge and go through the break. Either way you have set up the timing for a successful solo.

Of course, you can be too clever, and let a winning break go. Choose the players and shuffle the deck wisely.

When to Go

A break in the last lap or two can work, but it's awfully hard to make it stick— the pack speed is winding up, leadout riders and sprinters are at the front, and no one wants to let anything go.

About one-third of the race to go is an ideal time. Riders are no longer fresh, the early strong prime chasers and breakaway attempts have been caught, and other riders are not too fearful of a solo effort—they think there is still time and room to chase, yet the overall speed of the pack isn't so high that you can't get a good gap. I have seen most successful breaks work from this distance.

Get a Gap

You need at least 15 seconds quickly. Less than that and any fresh rider in the pack can close the gap, bridging or pulling, alone. If you're strong enough to make it stick, with a gap of more than 15 seconds the pack needs an organized effort.

If you've timed it right, the pack won't get organized for half a minute or so because you jumped when there was one of those natural lulls in the pack. If you don't have at least 15 seconds quickly, your chances of escape are not good.

Wind

Wind is your friend. Wind discourages a chase. If you are committed in the wind, your chances for success are greater because the pack is less likely to organize.

If the timing is right, it can be advantageous to attack on the tailwind side of the course. Just as the pack is getting organized, they'll hit the headwind side of the course and get delayed even further.

Commitment

Once you've put your cards on the table, make it stick. Get into time-trial mode. Be efficient around the corners. Ride at your anaerobic threshold or a little above. Go!

Criterium Solo Breakaway Heart Rate

Here's a heart-rate graph from a successful criterium solo breakaway. The race was 20 laps, each lap taking about 2 minutes. The solo effort began with a little more than 6 laps to go.

Figure 18–12

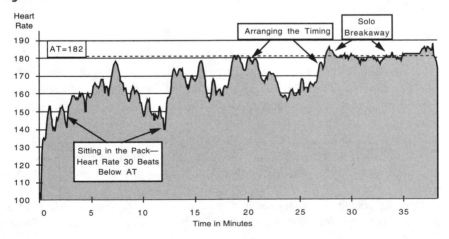

The more strong teammates you have, the better. If you have that crucial gap, and your teammates are sitting at the front, other riders will be discouraged from chasing.

Sometimes a couple of strong favorites will watch each other, the pack will watch them, and no chase will ensue. Perfect for you!

Even if it's a small race, with just family and friends around, a solo breakaway will get cheers. Spectators love to see a solo effort. Draw energy from the announcer and the crowd on each lap. Count down the laps with them. Stay focused.

Keep your pace, be committed. But watch what's happening behind you. If you are being caught by a small group, it's not over if you can stay with them. If you ease up a little and latch on, you can use them to keep you ahead of the field until the end of the race. They may even think you are so pooped that they let you not work and then, who knows, you might even take the breakaway sprint. So be aware of chasers.

It is also possible that by timing your efforts, you can splinter the chasers, and have solo riders chasing. It is more desirable to be pursued by a solo chaser since solo chasers are weaker than groups.

EGG ON YOUR FACE?

A solo breakaway attempt is often a gamble. If you win it's a great race. If you get caught, you may be too pooped to sprint and place. If you are strong, if the opportunity presents itself, and you have a chance, go for it! You won't know what you can do without trying and it's a lot more exciting than sucking wheel.

Prime Hunting

PRIMES DEFINED

Primes (pronounced *preems*) are prizes or awards given within a race. Most criterium riders are familiar with crit primes. The existence of these prizes may be known in advance, but their timing within the race often depends upon the whim of the race announcer, who will, say, announce a prime for the winner of the next lap.

Road races can have primes too. Prizes may be awarded to the first rider to the top of a hill. In circuit races, points may be awarded for several ascents, and the overall hilltop champion awarded "Queen of the Mountain" and a prize.

Over the course of a stage race it is usual to have a "King of the Mountains Winner," which is prestigious and valuable. Primes may be awarded on flatter sections as well. A separate jersey for a cumulative intermediate sprints winner may be awarded.

Races whose outcome is determined by primes or points are one of the most popular forms of track racing, called points races.

PRIME HUNTERS ARE DEVELOPED RIDERS

Prime hunting is a later facet of a local racer's development. When you first start racing and are inexperienced, your first priority is survival. This usually means doing as little work as possible and saving all your energy to last as long as you can in the race. It's foolish to waste energy in the middle of the race when it may jeopardize your ability to finish.

Once you can survive mass-start racing, the next step often is trying to finish the race in the lead bunch. Once you start placing you may start thinking about those primes.

PRIMES CAN BE VALUABLE

Prime hunting can be very lucrative in the 1,2's. Even in the lower categories and in the masters races the prizes received for prime hunting can be of greater value than those for many of the placings. Some riders may have a reasonable chance of winning primes and little chance of placing in large field sprints. They wisely concentrate their efforts on primes.

PRIME HUNTERS ARE FIT

Prime hunting provides another benefit: fitness. "The best training is racing," and the best race training may be prime hunting. Prime hunting raises your overall work level for the race and thereby helps you become fitter. It trains your body to withstand anaerobic efforts, and to recover from them.

Once you reach a certain level of fitness, if your only goal is placing in a crit, the race may be too easy. If you sit in until the finish, you will need to train harder than you race to keep fitness. If your goal is fitness for some larger goal, prime hunting may be valuable to that training. When you become an elite rider, you may race local races for every prime as well as the race win.

The heart-rate graphs which follow demonstrate what prime hunting requires and what prime hunting can do for training.

TWO HEART-RATE GRAPHS FROM DIFFERENT CRITS

The workout goal of the first crit, which had a short climb, was to place. This was successful. The workout goal of the second crit was anaerobic threshold (AT) training. This was also successful.

Figure 18–13

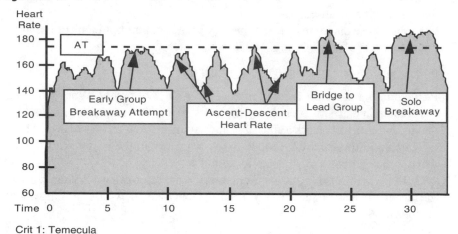

Crit 1: Temecula

Figure 18–14

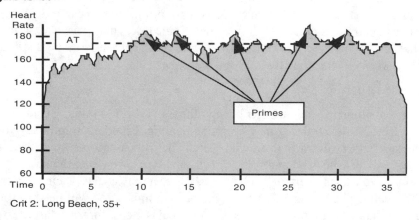

Crit 2: Long Beach, 35+

PRIME TRAINING BRINGS YOU CLOSER TO YOUR ANAEROBIC THRESHOLD

More time was spent around AT in the second race. The second crit was made into a harder crit by prime hunting. If the solo break of the first race had not been tactically right, and a field sprint had taken place, very little time would have been spent over AT. Fit riders may have difficulty in both placing and working hard in the same race.

TACTICAL CONSIDERATIONS

There are similarities and differences between successful prime hunters and successful race finishers.

Successful prime hunters may have less success in winning races. There is usually only a single rider who wins a prime. For this reason those out of contention tend to withdraw from the hunt early on. Contrast this to the sprint finish, where no one in contention gives way. For this reason a small gap or tactical surprise often succeeds in prime hunting where it does not at the end of a race.

Most primes are won with gaps on the field; most sprints are in bunches. Prime hunters usually do not want to waste their energy for second place. Race finishers often are thrilled for a second place.

Prime hunters do not need an excellent sprint. Race winners usually do. Prime hunters need a good sprint and excellent recovery. Race finishers need no recovery after the final sprint.

TEAMWORK EFFECTIVE IN PRIME HUNTING

Teamwork for primes can make prime hunting easy. Unlike the field sprint at the end of a race where everyone is going for it, there are relatively few in the field going for the primes.

The pace is very high in the finishing sprint, and a leadout may be vital. In prime hunting a teammate does as well to let his partner go, and merely jump on any chaser. A solo chaser with an opposing teammate on his wheel will often give up a prime: Either way he's likely a second at best. At the finish of a race a chance for second is well worth the effort.

PRIMES PRESENT TACTICAL OPPORTUNITIES WITHIN A RACE

Primes are opportunities. Opportunities are where things happen in races. Successful breakaways and attacks often develop just after or in concert with the gaps that occur on prime laps.

THANK YOU!

If your teammates help you win a prime, don't forget to acknowledge that help either by splitting points, by sharing the award, or with a simple thank you and post-race congratulations.

Leadouts

FASTEST DOES NOT ALWAYS WIN

It is not necessarily the fastest racer who wins the final sprint, or even wins the primes. Why is that?

One important reason is that the fastest sprinter may not be in the right place at the right time. She may get "boxed in." She may not be able to develop her sprint.

Or she may be forced to use her sprint at the wrong time (i.e., too early), with another rider taking advantage of her draft and coming around for the win.

TEAMMATE HELPS

A teammate can help considerably. Several can help even more.

It's easy to win the sprint if you are the fastest, and if you are third with 300 meters to go, second with 200 meters to go, and the way is clear to sprint. The problem is being in the right place.

A teammate can keep the pace high for you until the final 200 meters. A teammate can allow you to sit on her wheel until the last 200 meters, at which time you can come around your "leadout" woman.

TIMING

Timing is important. Your own leadout woman must not come to the front too soon. If she does, she might not be able to keep the speed high enough, and waves of riders may pass you on either side and your position may be lost.

TWO TEAMMATES

With two teammates to help, the first can pull the second to pull you. Then the leadout can begin earlier, and your position be assured more readily.

THREE TEAMMATES

With three teammates to help, you can have a sweeper on your wheel, a teammate who assures that no other rider takes advantage of you—the designated sprinter—and ensures that the team pulls you, but not your opponent, along.

SPRINTER DIRECTS

The designated sprinter directs the show. The leadout woman is at the front, and so can't see what is happening. She may need to be directed, told to go even faster, go left, or go right, to react to other challenges.

SUMMARY

- There must be at least one teammate to lead out the sprinter.
- The final leadout person drops off, after a maximal effort, 150–200 meters to the line.
- Watch out for waves that could "box in" your leadout.
- The sprinter directs.

Endgame: One-on-One

It has come down to the last part of the race, and you are away with one other rider. How do you plan the end of the race?

SECURE YOUR BREAK

Make some estimation of your opponent. If he is a decisively better time trialist and faster sprinter than you, it may be appropriate to acknowledge this and settle for second.

It may even be appropriate to tell him so. If he is uncertain of your abilities and starts to dicker with you about who should pull, putting you both at the risk of being caught by the pack or chase group, give the win away, be happy with second. And don't try to renege on your deal if you make one, or you'll never make another!

SET UP THE SPRINT

Normally, in a road sprint, it is easier to be behind your opponent with 250 meters to go. That way he leads you out and you jump and come around him with about 75 meters to go. If you have been trading pulls to stay away from the pack, you can psychologically set this up by pulling from about 400–500 meters to about 250 to go. That way it's "his turn." And save a little something with that last pull, if the pack isn't on you.

In a crit, decide ahead of time whether you want to lead out of the last turn, or if you want your opponent to do so. Set it up the way you want. For example, if it is 200 meters to the line after the turn, and there will be a tailwind, you probably want to lead it out to the finish line from the last corner. Arrange the last lap so your opponent pulls you toward the last corner and it's your turn to pull around the corner.

WATCH THE WIND

If there is a crosswind, set things up so that you'll have the faster leeward side.

CORRECT GEAR

Usually you have to shift a cog or two harder for the last sprint. You shift, keep a little slower cadence, then stand, jump, and wind it up.

CORRECT BODY POSITION

Don't forget: Hands in the drops, stand, accelerate to speed.

WHEN YOU GOTTA GO . . .

When you get to the point at which you can continuously accelerate to the finish line, it's time for you to go!

Endgame: Two-on-One

It has come down to the last part of the race, and you are away with two other riders. One is your teammate. How do you plan the finish?

SECURE YOUR BREAK

Two-on-one! Great! Either you or your teammate will probably win if you play your cards right.

Once you start working over your opponent, however, don't count on him ever working in this race with you again. Don't start dickering and playing until you reach the point in the race where either you or your teammate can successfully finish the race ahead of the chase group or pack alone!

DON'T BE GREEDY

What's the best that could happen? First and second for yourself and teammate. The worst? You get caught by the pack, or your opponent first, your teammate second, you third. Don't be greedy. If you are all about equal, try for first and second, sure, but be happy with a first and third, your teammate and you.

WHO IS THE BEST SPRINTER?

If your opponent is the best sprinter, you definitely do not want a sprint for first. If you are the strongest sprinter, you want your teammate to time-trial away for first, and you want to outsprint your opponent for second.

SET IT UP

There are many different ways to play it. Unless your opponent is by far the weakest sprinter, or concedes third, play it! Here are some examples:

PLENTY OF TIME UNTIL THE FINISH?

It is not necessarily the first attack that wins. Remember it may take many attacks to drop your opponent, or to get away. Or you may succeed only in weakening him.

Side to Side

Ride at a moderate pace, you on one side of the road, your teammate on the other. Who does the opponent stalk? The stalked rider slows down, the other speeds up.

The opponent is forced to jump and change sides, or your teammate is away for the win. When he switches sides, your teammate slows down and you speed up and jump both of them.

Your opponent must jump repeatedly twice as often as you and your teammate. If your opponent jumps you both, you and your teammate work together to chase him, then counterattack.

Back to Front

You are in a three-rider paceline. You and your teammate should pull only moderately.

- If your opponent is leading, the weaker teammate jumps as your opponent pulls off. If he chases, the stronger teammate sits on his wheel and counters the moment before catching.
- If your opponent is in second, and the pulling teammate is doing so only moderately, the rider in third can let a little gap open, jump into the slipstream gap to accelerate, and attack decisively.
- If the opponent is third, the second rider lets the first rider gap off and go away down the road, or rearranges the paceline.

NOT MUCH TIME UNTIL THE FINISH?

No time to dicker around because the pack or chasers threaten to catch you. You've got some choices:

Leadout

Weaker finisher leads out stronger teammate.

Gap

A stronger rider lets a gap open between himself and a teammate. If the opponent does not chase, the teammate wins. If an opponent does jump and chase, the strong rider is prepared to draft off the opponent and counterattack.

Body Language

Avoiding eye contact, crossing arms, smiling—body language tells us a lot about what another person is thinking. In the same way, observing the actions of other riders tells us a lot about what they can and cannot, might and might not, do on a bicycle.

RIDERS TELEGRAPH ATTACKS

- Shifting a gear combined with looking back almost always indicates an attack is imminent.
- Shifting hand position: Riders shifting hands to the drops may be planning an attack.
- Changing positions in the pack: Riders changing position in the pack may be planning something. Riders looking for a way out of a box in a group may be looking for an escape. Especially if giving up shelter to do so.

- Refastening shoe straps, or tightening them: An attack or hard effort is coming.
- Hitting the side of the hip: A signal from one rider to another that he's going to attack or give a leadout.
- Taking a few deep breaths may be used to mentally prepare some riders for an attack.
- Responding to jumps with snap: These are fresher riders.
- Tucking in a jersey or jacket: May be a signal of aerodynamic consciousness in planning an attack.
- Casting away water bottles: Many riders do it before climbs. Those who do so at other times may be planning an attack.
- Climbing at the front of the group: Riders who usually slip-slide on climbs but now are at the front may be planning to attack partway or at the top of the climb this time.
- Using a specialized piece of equipment: This may signal a rider's strategy, especially if different than their usual. An aerobar, 11 cog, or disc wheel may indicate a rider's plan for a proactive role in a race.

PICKING OUT TIRED OR WEAK RIDERS

- A rider looking down at his bottom bracket is usually tired.
- Loss of form, thrashing the upper body, shifting frequently, pedaling squares: These are all signs of a tired rider. Don't get trapped behind these riders or let these riders gap you off.
- Breathing a lot harder than you are usually means a person is working harder than you and may be dropped.
- Riders drinking early in a ride, and out of water early, without a feed/replacement may be tired later.
- Talkative riders become silent when tired.
- Riders who throw their bodies forward when climbing may be (especially if they are heavyset) track riders without climbing endurance.

INTERPRETATION REQUIRED

- Shifting gears: A rider shifting to a bigger gear may be planning an attack. If a rider shifts to a smaller one, it may mean that rider is tired.
- When a rider shifts during a climb, a bigger gear usually means that rider is strong; a smaller one may mean fatigue.
- Looking back can mean either a rider is tired and fearful of being caught or he wants to do only what's necessary to maintain a lead.
- A rider looking back from a small group may be thinking about launching an attack from the small group, or may be waiting for a bridging teammate.

- Two riders talking together may indicate their willingness to attack or work together.

DANGEROUS RIDERS

- Riders cutting each other off, or returning foul language and behaviors, may signal a dangerous situation. You need to avoid those riders.
- Riders who can't hold a straight line when they shift gears or drink from their water bottles.
- Riders who don't hold a straight line at any time.

Lulling Your Opponents into a False Sense of Security

WHAT WE'RE TALKING ABOUT

You want to ride away from your rivals in a race. If you say to them: "I want to ride up the road, let me go," what do you think they'd say in return? "No way. We'd prefer that you stay with us."

Suppose you say: "Well, I am a little stronger than you, so please let me go." They might say: "Stronger or not, we'll fight to stay in your slipstream and keep you with us."

The problem is that, psychologically, you may have approached this situation all wrong.

Suppose, instead, you say: "I'm really no stronger than all of you. You can catch me any time you like. Let me sit out there and cook alone awhile. Then, when you feel like it, you can gobble me up and make me look foolish." Your rivals are likely to say: "Sure. Go fry."

THE DANGLE

There's a critical time gap in lots of crit racing. About 15 seconds. Less than a 15-second gap and a single, determined rider can chase you down. More than 15 seconds and it usually takes a concerted effort to catch.

Suppose you sit out about 10 seconds. If you don't seem to be making any progress, the pack often doesn't care that much. They know that anytime they want, they can come up and get you.

It's a paradox. If you work harder, they'll start chasing. Keep the same distance and they are content.

So keep the same distance and lull them into a false sense of security. Now, at a turn or curve in the road, really punch it. Now you've got more than 30 seconds on the pack and may even be out of sight.

The leaders in the pack may be surprised—they can't imagine that you've escaped. Others may think you have been caught. Even if you can be seen, now the gap is too large for an individual to bridge and so a chase is less likely.

This also works on hills. Break away and dangle just 15 seconds up the road. The group figures: "He's not too far ahead, we'll catch him on the descent." After settling the group into this dangle scenario, start *really* working. The group, set in their rhythm, will still believe they can catch you. They've become convinced that you are "just there," even though you've actually left them far behind.

WE COULD ALWAYS CHASE HIM DOWN

How often have you heard riders say: "We stayed with every attack, until the very last one." Of course. They succeeded until they failed.

Attack a number of times, without complete commitment, at less than maximum pace. Let yourself be caught.

If you attack half-heartedly a few times, and you get caught pretty easily, your rivals may get lazy and let out your leash a little.

The one time they fail to respond, you go, but this time you're committed.

THE COUNTERPUNCH

Someone else is forcing the race. This rider is saying "I am the strongest." He attacks repeatedly, you let the group respond. You respond with submaximum efforts. The group catches. You seem to be just hanging on.

Now make an apparently wild attack yourself. The group thinks you can't keep it up. Besides, they are all watching the strongman.

But you are strong. And you do keep it up.

CHAPTER 19

Time Trialing

Time Trials Defined

A time trial is a timed bicycling event. Time trials are almost always individual events. It's one rider against the clock. Often called the "race of truth," the time trial is often perceived as the ultimate test of a cyclist's ability.

In multi-day events, the individual time-trial stages are usually crucial to a rider's overall success.

Riders are usually started at 30- to 60-second intervals.

A team time trial is a timed event for a group of riders. All riders on the team start at the same time. The time is determined after a specified number of members of the group finish.

No drafting is allowed except within a team. Common distances are 10 miles and 25 miles (40K) for individual events, and up to 100 km for team events. On the track, distances from 200 to 5,000 meters are standard. Special considerations apply to these events.

Almost all great bicycle racers have been great time trialists. Although time trials are a specific form of bicycle racing, the ability to time-trial is an important element in many mass-start bicycling events: The ability to maintain a solo or small break, the ability to bridge (leave one group and join another up the road), the ability to chase back to the pack after a flat tire or other mechanical problem, or the ability to solo to victory—all involve time-trial skills.

Time trialing is also the essential feature of other forms of racing. For example, mountain bike racing is essentially a time trial off-road. Ultra-distance cycling events, such as the Race Across America, are long individual time trials. The bike leg of a triathlon is a time trial.

Since pack skills are not required, time trialing is often an excellent place for new riders to assess their potential.

Whether a new rider or a seasoned veteran, time trialing is so important in bicycle racing that I'll discuss this aspect in detail.

Even if you are more interested in criteriums or road races, reading about how this bicycling discipline can be analyzed, dissected, and learned will serve as an example for other forms of racing.

Five Components of Time Trials

Time trials have five important aspects:

1. Physical requirements
2. Technique
3. Pre- and post-race preparation
4. Mental attitude
5. Equipment

Each of these aspects will be discussed in turn. I'll then discuss team time trialing, pacing, and the effect of altitude on time trials.

PHYSICAL ABILITY

Strength

You need strength in your legs and buttocks for successful time trialing. Pushing a big gear for 1 hour is much different from racing a crit or riding a club ride for the same period of time. The gluteal (butt) muscles are used to a much greater extent. It is common for inexperienced time trialists to be sore in their gluts for days after a 40K TT. It is common for occasional time trialists to not be able to walk normally for several hours.

Practice time trialing in "the position" at full power to strengthen these muscles. Excellent time trialists never get out of the "aero" position on flat courses. Physical adaptation to this position requires that you ride in this position frequently.

Don't forget to stretch those gluts.

Aerobic Capacity

You need aerobic ability. You want to increase your anaerobic threshold. You can't increase your maximum heart rate—that's genetically determined. You are looking to increase the percentage of maximum heart rate you can sustain.

Fit time trialists generally ride at 92±2% of their maximum heart rate for 1 hour. This applies to events held at moderate temperatures and at sea level.

Interval training is important in developing this ability. It is better to practice going 1 mile as fast as you can five times than it is to go 10 miles once. Intervals of 2 to 4 minutes serve the all-round road rider and time trialist very well.

Time trialists probably need sustained efforts of 20 minutes or so every week. These efforts can be achieved in races or group rides as well as individually on the road or stationary trainer.

Be sure to read the sections on aerobic training and heart-rate training in Chapters 9 and 10.

TECHNIQUE

Train Specifically

The techniques and bike-handling skills required to successfully pilot a front disc or three-spoke wheel and forearm-support bars are specific to time trialing. Train specifically by practicing and riding in the aero position with the equipment you will use on race day.

Starting Gear

At the start, you normally have your chain in the big ring. You start in an easy cog, but not the easiest—or the chain angle will be extreme and your chain may skip with your start. If the chain angle is too great you also risk derailment if you pedal backwards to get your cranks positioned. Ride in your starting gear for at least a few hundred yards before the start to make sure you have shifted precisely into gear.

Set Your Watch

If you are using a stopwatch, set it off 1 minute before you start. This way you'll be able to time yourself but not have to reach for the start button of your watch when you should have both your hands in the drops to launch off the start line.

Crank Position at the Start

With your hands in the drops, leg positioned for the first downstroke at 10 o'clock, and arms and wrists straight, squeeze your brakes and rise out of your saddle with a second or two to go, pull up with the pedals, remember to breathe, and you're off!

Pacing

A specific section on pacing theory is found later in this chapter. Consider a pacing strategy.

Accelerate to speed quickly, but not beyond your aerobic maximum. You should be working at your anaerobic threshold the entire event. When you reach the finish, if you have a spring left, you have not worked hard enough during the time trial!

On flat, windless courses, excellent time trialists have fairly equal splits for the first and last halves. If your time for the first half is slower than the second by more than 30 seconds, you probably did not warm up enough. If your second half is slower, you may have a problem with mental attitude, pacing, or endurance.

In practice, notice your heart rate and effort with about 3 miles to go. This is probably the heart rate and effort you should be riding from the beginning. Notice your effort more than your heart rate. Without a super warm-up it may take 5 to 10 minutes to achieve this cruising anaerobic threshold heart rate. With rare exceptions, do not exceed this level until the last 5 minutes or less of the race.

An exception to exceeding your threshold is a rolling or hilly course. It is reasonable to float a little before a climb and then slightly exceed your anaerobic threshold as you ascend to avoid losing momentum up a hill or roller. Floating doesn't mean you stop working. Do not let your heart rate drop more than 5 beats per minute. Slight anaerobic effort does not mean sprinting—it means you may exceed your threshold by a maximum of 5 beats. No more!

Cadence

Optimal cadence is between 75 and 95 rpm for most riders under most circumstances.

Position

Position on the bike is the most important aerodynamic factor. Having your back flatter and head lower by as little as 5 millimeters may be more important than trick wheels.

In order to achieve good position, most riders need to move their saddles a little forward, raise them to compensate, and lengthen their effective stem length.

Head Up

Ride with your head up. It's safer. It's also more aerodynamic. Many riders erroneously believe that they are more aerodynamic with their heads down. Watch other riders. Notice that with the head looking down the back of the helmet pops up and the smooth transition of airflow across to the back is lost.

Aerobar Position

Priorities for positioning with forearm-support bars are:

1. Elbows close together
2. Back flat
3. Chin tucked in, in line with wrists
4. Knee pedaling style close to top tube

Look for the Fast Lane

Most roads have a "best place to ride." In choosing where you are going to ride, consider safety, shortest line, and surface. The fastest place to ride is usually a couple of feet in from the edge of the lane—where the inside wheels of most cars have made the pavement a little bit smoother and a little bit faster.

Hugging the shoulder of the road may be the safest location only if there is a lot of traffic on the course. The shoulder usually has the most glass and other debris, making it the most likely place for a flat.

With an organized event, signs warn motorists of your presence and riding down the middle of the lane is not dangerous.

Practice Starts and Turnarounds

There is a certain amount of technique for the start and for the turn. Practicing five intervals with five starts and five turnarounds is recommended rather than a single longer effort as a way to build your physical ability and technique.

The turn is best performed asymmetrically. You want to save breaking for the last moment. Slowly coasting into the turn wastes time. Ride a couple of meters beyond the turnaround along the right edge of the road. Make an acute turn and get back up to speed quickly. This method is slightly longer than a symmetric curve, but allows for better control of the bike and a quicker start back up to speed.

Legal Drafting

Vehicles passing you may provide momentary draft. There is nothing illegal about edging to the center of the road and slightly picking up the pace to momentarily draft them. Vehicles traveling toward you may slow you down. You may wish to move toward the gutter to avoid their headwind draft.

Dry Mouth

Dry mouth is a common problem for time trialists. You mouth is dried by all that hard breathing. You can increase saliva flow by riding with your tongue touching the roof of your mouth.

PRE- AND POST-RACE PREPARATION

Tapering

Tapering before an important time trial usually involves reducing mileage, but not intensity, a couple of weeks before the big event. Reduce mileage about one-third. Two days before the event I hardly ride at all. For out-of-town races, this is my travel day.

Ride the Course Ahead of Time

The pre-race ritual includes riding the course for familiarization. Ideally, you will ride the course the day before your event, at the same time as your event. This will allow you to judge wind, temperature, and other factors.

Preliminary Warm-up, 30 Minutes

You must start the time trial warmed up. It is not unreasonable to warm up for 1 hour.

Have two warm-ups. In the first, preliminary warm-up, ride to the start line and synchronize your watch to the official clock. Check and make sure the officials say they will start on time; if the competition is already in progress, make sure it is on schedule.

If competition is in progress, note the length of time after officials call a rider to the line that that rider actually starts. In some time trials officials call riders 10 or more minutes before starting. You then know you don't necessarily have to come running when you hear your number called!

Ride away from the course and parked vehicles to find a suitable area for more intense work. Find a place close enough to be aware of what is going on, but secluded enough for concentration.

Perhaps take off a layer of clothing and drink a bottle of glucose water (e.g., sports drink or half-strength apple juice).

Figure 19–1

Preliminary Warm-up Summary	• Easy—Heart rate less than 70% of maximum.
	• Check start location.
	• Check finish location.
	• Check start times.
	• Check schedule.
	• Check official clock, synchronize computer/watch.
	• Check time from "the call" to actual start.

Intense Warm-up, 30 Minutes

The most controlled and best warm-ups are on stationary trainers. This is vital if it is cold or raining.

Intensive warm-up includes several hard efforts. No sprints or jumps, however. No anaerobic efforts.

A time-trial warm-up schedule is found below. The heart-rate and power percentages are approximate. Their correlation will depend upon the trainer setup and your physiology. Not all riders will be able to spin at a cadence of 120 rpm.

Warm up to time-trial heart rate in a gear easier than the one you will power during the TT. Rest a minute, drink a little.

In TT gearing, warm up to TT pace.

Heart rate will not reach the suggested levels until near the end of each

Figure 19–2 **Intense Warm-Up—30 Minutes**

Time	Heart Rate (% of max)	Gear	Cadence (rpm)	Power (% of TT)	Notes
2 minutes	70	Moderate	90	50	
2	75		100	55	
2	80		110	60	
2	90		120	70	*TT HR, but less effort*
2 *Rest*					
3	75	Hard	80	85	
3	85		85	90–95	
3	90		90	100	*TT HR and effort*
2 *Rest*					
3	70	Moderate	85	50	
3	90		110+	70	*TT HR, but less effort*
3	70		80	<50	

interval. Don't try to get your heart rate up to the suggested level as soon as you begin each interval—you will be working too hard.

Without a stationary trainer, a favorite technique is to be a mile or two from the start and pretend you are late. Time-trial to the start with almost full effort.

Arrive no more than 5 minutes before your scheduled start time.

Ergogenic Aids

Pre-race warm-up may include a few aspirins and some caffeine about 1 hour before the start. Controlled studies evaluating the use of aspirin and caffeine before time trials are lacking, but anecdotal evidence supports their use. After warm-up, have a few ounces of fluid at the start line.

Helper at the Start

Ideally you'll have a helper near the line to give you a half bottle of water or dilute carbohydrate solution. You'll be able to leave your warm-up jacket or other items with your helper without having to search for your car parked some distance from the line.

Post-race Immediate Help

Post-race preparation includes instructing your helper to be located several hundred meters beyond the finish line to hand you a warming jacket, sponge or face cloth, two bottles of fluids, and some low-fat carbohydrate food.

Post-race Headache Recovery

With a full 40K effort you can expect post-time-trial headache. After cleaning up back in your room, have something more to eat and perhaps a few more aspirins too. You may wish only to spin and ride briefly a day or two after a hard 40K time trial. It may take a week to recover completely from your effort.

Evaluate Performance

After your time trial, evaluate your performance. Consider the contents of this section and see where you did well and where you might improve.

MENTAL ATTITUDE

By establishing a pre- and post-race ritual as just discussed, you will be more mentally focused and relaxed. Focus, without undue anxiety, improves performance.

The Difference May Be Mental

The mind is important. Riders of equal strength do not ride the same times. Some riders finish a time trial too fresh and able to ride more. Others are totally exhausted and need to recover. The ability to go your hardest and know that you are pushing absolutely as hard as you can requires experience and the motivation to perform. It's common to hear riders say they are not tired enough and could have ridden harder.

- Visualization techniques can help. Read about visualization in Chapter 24.
- A cycling computer or heart-rate monitor helps some riders.
- Set yourself attainable goals and keep track of your progress.
- At least monthly time-trial practice allows you to learn your limits.

Mental Tricks

- Count as you stroke. Count odd numbers or half reps so that you alternate left and right leg emphasis with your counting. Counting each stroke of my left and right legs, I personally like counting in reps of 5, with slightly extra force on the 1st and 3rd counts.
- Ask yourself if you can go harder. Go harder.
- Notice the regularity of your breathing. A short while after you start you'll find you are taking a breath for every so many pedal strokes. Breathe just a little faster. Your pedal strokes will go a little faster to keep the rhythm.
- Don't think about how bad you feel. Think instead about how good it feels to be working hard, how regular your breathing is. See yourself posting your goal time, visualize yourself being patted on the back or getting your reward.

EQUIPMENT

Equipment May Matter

If you are gauging your progress, rating yourself against yourself, you can ride the same equipment month after month and the fancy stuff doesn't really matter. The aero stuff matters most for those who are racing against others, not themselves.

An aero bike all tricked-out isn't a priority for a 25-year-old male who rides 10 miles in 35 minutes. Money need not be invested so much as time in training. For a 65-year-old woman with that time, like Margaret Nolan, aero equipment is crucial to being the best in the country.

Purists Don't Ride as Fast

Some "purists" decry the cost of special time-trial equipment. The fact is most of the equipment is not much costlier than bicycling gear in general, and if you want to be competitive, you need the tools of the trade.

Time-trial with and without equipment. See the difference. When you become competitive, it makes no sense to put considerable effort into training, expense into travel, and sacrifice in free time and income from work only to go several minutes slower than you would with the right equipment.

Don't Ride New Equipment on Race Day

Riders frequently make the error of using new equipment for the first time in competition. Riders get excited about the possibility of going faster with the latest gizmo and purchase or borrow equipment just before a race. Since some equipment is specialized, riders often save it for race day, only to encounter small problems during the race. Although time-trial equipment is vital, leave time to test equipment thoroughly under race conditions before competition.

Use the aero stuff, yes, but rely on the tried-and-true and test your equipment well in advance. Before a time trial be sure to test your equipment with full power and speed. Problems such as chain-freewheel incompatibility or an insufficiently tightened skewer may not surface with less than full effort.

Freewheel Selection

You need a straight block. You don't want to find yourself with a gear choice that is too hard or too easy. Get a 12/13/14/15/16/17/x/x 7- or 8-speed. Choose your chain rings to match your ability.

Chain Ring Selection

The standard big chain ring on a standard road bike has 52 or 53 teeth. Most of us leave well enough alone. If you're a lot faster or a lot slower, or a time-trial specialist, replace the standard with the custom using the following guidelines:

On a flat, windless course, if you ride a 60-minute 40K TT (slow for senior elite men) you need a 50-tooth ring. For every 1 to 2 minutes of difference, change your chain ring size by one tooth. Ride 63 minutes? Use a 48 ring. Ride 55 minutes? Use a 53 ring. Riding a tandem in 48 minutes? You need a 58. If there is wind or a downhill, you need more gear.

Be Prepared with a Big Gear

You must be adequately geared. You don't want to be coasting downhill or spinning 120 rpm with a terrific tailwind. Since time trials are often held in rural areas, away from traffic congestion, they usually have some wind. Be prepared! I have ridden several 40K time trials in less than 20 minutes in one direction and more than 40 in the other. The fastest time trialists in this country push a 55/12 on windless courses. I have ridden time trials with a terrific tailwind, where even a massive 60/11 has not been enough!

Position First

The biggest piece of aerodynamic machinery is your body. Position on the bike is the most important aerodynamic factor.

Aerodynamic Equipment

Fast wheels, aero-bars, an aero-helmet, and a skinsuit are the most important wind-cheaters.

Remove your pump and spare tire bag. If you get a flat you don't stand a chance. If it is a flat course, you don't need an inner chain ring or a front shift lever. Removing the front derailleur, however, risks derailment.

For time trials under an hour, you don't need a water bottle or its cage. Usually you are working too hard to get the fluid down, or don't want to take the time to drink. Riding with a water bottle is not only a weight and aerodynamic error, it is a distraction.

Aero V-shaped rims are faster than box rims. Fewer spokes are faster than many. Too few spokes risks wheel failure and handling instability. Bladed and radial front spokes give modest advantages if the wheel is well built.

Narrow tires, at most 3 millimeters wider than the rim, are faster than wider tires. Flimsy narrow tires risk punctures for heavy riders.

Disc wheels are faster than almost all other types of wheels. On the front, they are very difficult to control. Heavy solid wheels are a disadvantage on uphill time trials. Wheel covers don't work. Some three-spoked wheels may be faster than discs in crosswinds.

There's a knack to pinning on numbers to minimize their aerodynamic resistance. Alone at a race, use your car's steering wheel to give shape to and support your jersey or skinsuit. An advanced attachment method is to use a spray adhesive, such as 3M's ReMount or Super 77, to perfectly position and adhere your number.

Mechanical and Road Resistance

Lubrication is vital. A well-lubricated chain can save half a minute over a poorly maintained one. A loose chain helps reduce chain friction; a very loose chain risks derailment.

Some riders use oil in their bearings, instead of grease, and if the bearings are sealed, remove the seals. I am not sure messing with your bearings is a good idea. There is a difference between bearing friction on the bikestand and friction with load. I am not sure using oil accomplishes anything.

Wheels are not weight balanced—the valve stem hole and valve stem unbalance most wheels. When allowed to move freely, from the heavier side up, they oscillate until the heavier side is down. Wheels should oscillate at least seven times when clamped by their quick releases or bolts either on the bike or in a truing stand. Many hub bearing binding problems are uncovered only when under the load of quick release or bolted tension. Testing the freedom of your wheel bearings must be done under load.

Tires that can take higher pressures and are pumped to 160–180 pounds lower road resistance. This means using sew-ups.

Longer cranks can be more efficient for straight time trials.

Weight is of little importance in steady speed, flat time trials. If the course has hills or is rolling, weight becomes a factor to consider. On an uphill time trial, every pound can be worth 20 seconds in every hour of the event.

Team Time Trialing

The idea is to allow a predetermined number of the group to finish together in as fast a time as possible.

TEAM TIME-TRIAL SETUP

Here's a scenario: You have six people in your team. You need to finish at least four out of the six—you are allowed to have two team members drop out. This may be because they are not as strong, or because of a mechanical problem.

Let us assume the course is varied terrain. What are some important points to keep in mind?

SMOOTHNESS

Foremost in importance: You or someone else on the team will be riding at your maximum. After all, if no one on the team is at their max, the group is not going as fast as it can.

This means that it is vital that the group be smooth and consistent in its energy output. The rider coming to pull at the front must not accelerate. He must pull smoothly forward while the retiring rider drops back by ever so slightly decreasing his output.

ENERGY OUTPUT

Since some riders are stronger than others, it seems reasonable that some riders will pull harder (at a greater speed) than others. This is not the best technique. It's not pulling harder that is required, it is pulling longer. As already expressed, the weakest rider must be at a maximum time-trial output throughout. The strongest rider must not exceed the weakest rider's anaerobic threshold. Stronger riders pull longer, not faster.

RIDER SPACING

At first, riders might think that the most efficient spacing would be to have stronger riders alternate with weaker ones in the paceline order. As it turns out, this is one of the most inefficient ways to succeed in a team time trial.

Why?

1. The hardest parts about working a paceline come when it is your turn to pull and when you reattach to the back of the moving paceline after you've taken your pull and pulled off.
2. You get a better draft when drafting behind two riders than behind one.

A hard place to be is behind the strongest rider of a paceline. You have to take a pull after the strongest rider. Since a single rider provides less draft than the group, you get the least rest behind the strongest rider and then you have to pull! You rest the least. If you have a strong rider behind you, it will also be harder to reattach to the paceline after your pull.

Therefore, if you are a weak rider and you are nestled between the two strong riders in a four-person line, you are in for it!

It usually works out much better to have the second-strongest rider behind the strongest one—then the strongest rider has to reattach when the next-strongest rider is pulling.

Modifications may be necessary when rider size is considered.

HILLY TIME-TRIAL COURSE

The weakest riders have to save their strength much more so than on a flat course, to enable them to climb reasonably well with the group. The weakest riders of the group may actually never pull on the flats, in order to have the best chance of staying with the group on the climbs.

EQUALIZE YOUR CONTRIBUTION

If during the race you can climb more comfortably than the designated fastest or strongest riders of the group, things are not proportioned correctly. When it comes to the flat, either you need to do more work to equalize your contribution or the "strongest" needs to pull less.

KNOW YOUR LIMITS

Weaker riders of the group must know their limits. Sometimes they must sit just off the back of the rotating team paceline and let the other riders pull.

Pacing

It's your district track championships. You are riding the 3-kilometer time trial. Your target time is 4 minutes, 17 seconds. At what speed should you ride?

You are riding your district 40K time trial. Your personal record is 61 minutes. You believe you can break an hour. Assuming a flat out-and-back course with no wind, at what pace should you ride?

WHY PACE?

Figuring out at what pace you should ride is crucial to great performance. The difference between going out too hard and pacing yourself can cost you 10 seconds in a 3K and a minute in 10 miles.

PROVE THE VALUE OF PACING

It is easy to prove the importance of pacing, on your own, with a simple test.

Read Chapters 12 and 13 on trainer workouts and experiment with isolated leg training if you haven't already done so. After several weeks of isolated leg training on the trainer, you will have dialed in the gears that let you push about 55 rpm for 4 minutes.

SLOW VS. FAST START

Let us assume that you find the perfect gear for which 55 rpm is the most you can push for 4 minutes. After several weeks, try this experiment: Ride a cadence of 53 for the first 2 minutes, then 57 for the last 2 minutes. At your next workout session, try riding at a cadence of 57 for the first 2 minutes and 53 for the last 2 minutes.

Which way was harder? The vast majority of riders find the slow-start strategy much easier.

51/49 PRINCIPLE

Recent scientific reports confirm that going at about 98% race pace the first half and 102% race pace the second half is the best strategy. That is, the first half takes about 51% of elapsed time, the second half 49%.

If you are shooting for 4:17 in 3 kilometers, that is 257 seconds. On a 333-meter track, and subtracting 5 seconds for the start, you need a 252-second pace for nine laps. That's 28 seconds a lap.

Let's ignore the first and second laps—their times are different because the start and acceleration to speed make them special.

A suitable strategy would be to ride up to half a second slower than 28 seconds per lap the third and fourth laps, and a half or more second faster than last laps. This strategy has been borne out in numerous championship pursuit rides.

PACING LONGER RIDES

The longer the ride, the closer the overall half splits are to 50/50. A 40K championship TT might have nearly even splits. If the 40K were to be divided into 4-kilometer tenths, however, the first tenth might be at 49% race pace, and the last tenth at 51%. This means that most of the race might be paced at 6 minutes per 4 kilometers. The first 4K might be paced 5 to 10 seconds slower, the last 4K that much faster.

WHY PACING WORKS

A simplistic physiologic explanation of the pacing principle may be the following:

Go out too slowly and you never have the time to catch up.

Go out too fast and your lactic acid levels zoom too quickly.

It is easier to tolerate high lactic acid levels for short periods of time rather than longer ones.

If high lactic acid levels must be endured, it is easier to tolerate them at the end rather than at the beginning of a race.

Psychologically, the natural tendency of many athletes is to get excited at big competitions and go out too hard. By consciously backing off just a little this risk is reduced. Build to a crescendo rather than starting with a bang and fizzling.

Effect of Altitude on Time Trials

Altitude improves performance for flat time-trial events, no matter what the distance. The aerodynamic benefit of reduced air pressure more than compensates for the reduced oxygen available for energy production.

REDUCED OXYGEN VS. IMPROVED AERODYNAMICS

It is no surprise that track cycling events, which rely upon a large contribution of anaerobic energy production, are performed more quickly at altitude.

This is also the case in running events under 400 meters. Longer events in running are performed more slowly at altitude, because reduced air for aerobic metabolism slows the racer more than reduced air resistance helps aerodynamics.

ALTITUDE LOWERS TIME-TRIAL HEART RATE

You cannot work as hard at altitude as you can at sea level. Hence, time-trial threshold heart rate will be lower.

Time trialing is a balance between aerobic capacity and leg strength. Bigger gears lower heart rate. Since aerobic capacity is reduced at altitude, a bigger gear is favored. This further lowers heart rate.

If you know your sea-level threshold heart rate, it is helpful to understand and expect a reduction at altitude. Riders who monitor their heart rates and do not expect decreases may find that they pace incorrectly, going out too hard and trying to achieve the impossible.

VO$_2$ MAX REDUCTION

VO$_2$ max is a measure of the maximum amount of oxygen that the body can use to produce energy. VO$_2$ max is reduced at altitude.

Several models for the reduction in VO$_2$ exist. François Perronnet and others from the University of Montreal have helped develop the fourth column in the following table.

Table 19-1 **VO₂ Max Reduction at Altitude**

Altitude (meters)	Altitude (feet)	Pressure (mm Hg)	VO₂ Max (% sea level)
0	0	760	100.0
500	1,640	716	98.1
1,000	3,281	674	96.4
1,500	4,921	634	94.6
2,000	6,562	596	92.5
3,000	9,843	530	86.0
3,500	11,483	493	83.1
4,000	13,123	462	78.0

DEMONSTRATED EFFECTS OF ALTITUDE ON HEART RATE

Review the heart-rate graphs that follow from the records of the Senior Nationals in Dublin, Ohio, the Record Challenge Time Trial at Moriarty, New Mexico, and the Colorado District Championships in Alamosa. They are all performed by the same rider. The essential feature to note is how, with increasing altitude, this athlete's threshold heart rate falls.

Figure 19–3 **Tandem race time trial, Dublin, Ohio. Altitude: 780 feet.**

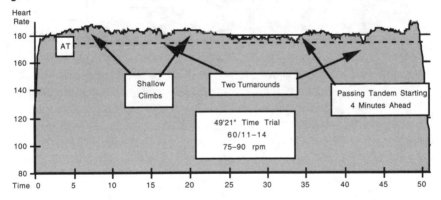

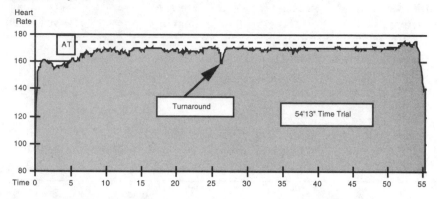

Figure 19–4 **Tandem race time trial, Moriarty, New Mexico. Altitude: 6,215 feet.**

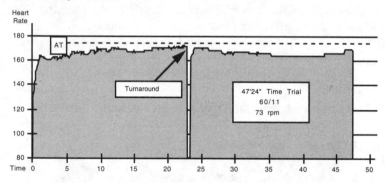

Figure 19–5 **Tandem race time trial, Alamosa, Colorado. Altitude: 7,550 feet.**

Part Five

CYCLING IN YOUR HEAD

CHAPTER 20

Motivation

Although riders may wish it were different, you don't buy motivation at the store and take a pill of it in the morning. By understanding what makes you tick and why you're doing what you're doing, you may improve your performance.

What We're Talking About

Motivation is the ability to focus on a goal and work toward that goal with all your effort, regardless of physical ability. It has two important elements: direction—the choice of goal; and intensity—how energized the individual is toward that goal. Intensity, which is related to psychic energy, is influenced by emotion.

Intrinsic and Extrinsic Motivation

Motivation of an individual may come from within (intrinsic) or from without (extrinsic).

People who are intrinsically motivated have an inner striving to be successful, to master their task, to reach their goal. Athletes who are intrinsically motivated participate because they love the sport. Intrinsic rewards—such as feelings of accomplishment, mastery, or self-confidence—tend to be self-perpetuating and powerful.

Extrinsic motivation comes from other people through positive and negative reinforcement. Positive reinforcers increase the likelihood or frequency of positive behaviors; negative reinforcers decrease the likelihood of positive behaviors.

Positive reinforcers—the carrots—include praise, trophies, recognition, and money.

Negative reinforcers—the sticks—include ridicule, embarrassment, and punishment.

Most athletes are motivated by a combination of intrinsic and extrinsic rewards, although the proportions may vary greatly.

Extrinsic rewards that are excessive or manipulating, and those that are not contingent upon accomplishment, tend to lose effectiveness. Extrinsic rewards can also increase or decrease intrinsic motivation. With time, many extrinsic rewards lose their value: Enough prizes, trophies, or money will eventually fail to motivate. When earned for accomplished behavior, extrinsic rewards can be extremely motivating. Extrinsic rewards that transform into intrinsic rewards tend to sustain motivation.

Motivation Theories

HIERARCHY OF NEEDS

On the most basic of levels, we need to satisfy our hunger, thirst, sleep, and sex drives. After that, we look to our safety and security needs.

Once our basic needs are satisfied, we seek to satisfy our social needs for belonging, love, self-esteem, self-worth, and self-respect. We also have needs for play, excitement, and avoiding boredom.

Older athletes may be motivated by the perceived retention of youth and health that exercise may impart.

OPTIMAL CHALLENGE/FRUSTRATION

An optimal challenge or frustration results in the greatest motivation. Too much challenge or frustration—a task too difficult—reduces motivation. Too little challenge or frustration—a task too easy—also reduces motivation.

CONTROL

We have relatively little control over our genetic ability or talent, the demands of a given race, and luck. We have relatively more control over our own effort and preparation.

Many athletes correctly attribute their success to effort and preparation; they often incorrectly attribute their failure to factors over which they have little control.

Why We Race

Our motivation to ride or race may come from reinforcers, needs, or challenges.

Most of us race for one or more of the following reasons:

- "Fun," which involves stimulation, excitement, challenge, and creativity.
- Health and fitness.
- Social affiliation with others, belonging to and being accepted by a group.
- Self-worth, confirmed by demonstrating competency.

These reasons all satisfy social needs. For some professional riders, it's more a question of economics and earning a living.

FUN

Stimulation must not be too much or too little. The skill difficulty must match ability. There must be challenge and some success. Realistic goals are needed. Control of the scheduling of activities and events, and not always having "to perform," keeps things fun.

HEALTH AND FITNESS

Bicycle racing helps many improve and maintain their health and fitness.

Bicycling injuries are common. If you race only for health and fitness, crashes in rainy, tightly cornered criteriums may soon cause you to leave the sport.

SOCIAL AFFILIATION

An appropriate group is necessary. You need to be able to identify with your team and be accepted by teammates.

If you are a junior rider in a masters club, it may be difficult to maintain motivation unless other important needs are met.

SELF-WORTH

Self-worth, self-esteem, confidence, and achievement are closely tied. Goals appropriate to ability levels help maintain motivation. Competency, mastery, and success will be important.

Suppose you are a 32-year-old racer, beginning bicycle racing after a successful running career ended by injury. You are used to placing in 10K races.

But bike racing is different. Different muscles are used, different skills are required, and different tactics are employed. You may have difficulty with self-worth if you start out racing against the Category 1, 2 masters. Start racing senior Cat 4, 5, or masters 3, 4, 5. Your feelings of self-worth are less likely to be affronted. As you master your level, advance.

Getting Motivated

- Understand your reinforcers and needs—why you ride, why you race.
- Set realistic, specific goals.
- Expect to be frustrated at first, or limit task difficulty.
- Get coaching or advice as a way to find the most efficient, direct, and intense reinforcers.
- Set up appropriate reinforcers.
- Work on the most controllable factors—preparation and effort.
- Get confident.
- Achieve your goals.

CHAPTER 21

Avoiding Burnout

Burnout Examples

Were you all gung ho at the beginning of the year, just itching to start racing, and wondering why there aren't races all year round—whereas now you could take it or leave it if there was a race this weekend? Did you ever find yourself signed up for a race, but when it came time to pack things up in the morning, you didn't really want to look at your bike? Ever find yourself having planned a workout a couple of weeks in advance when you were so hot to structure workouts and get stronger only to find that when the time came, you wanted to do something else? Or, having gone hard the last couple of weeks, have you found it difficult even to get psyched up enough to go out on the club ride?

Well, maybe you're suffering from burnout, something most seasoned bike racers know all too well.

Causes of Burnout

Burnout comes from doing too much. The "too much" is usually too much on your bike, but sometimes it's too much in the rest of your life. If you've developed a good training schedule and then your family comes visiting and stays with you, you'll have less time. You may find yourself rushing your workouts and lacking enthusiasm.

Usually burnout is from pushing "the edge" too hard. Sometimes you know you've been working hard, and might understand why you are tired. Sometimes it may be less clear.

The solution is usually to cut down on your riding.

Racers Beware

Burnout affects racers more than recreational riders because racers tend to push themselves harder. For example: You usually ride the club ride, which is about 35 miles, on Saturday, and ride 50 miles on Sunday with the women's team. Tuesday is usually your sprint day, and Wednesday a long hard endurance day.

One Saturday you race 60 instead of your usual moderate 35 miles. And you ride your hard Sunday ride. It's easy to see why you'll not feel like doing your usual 10 sprints on Tuesday or that you'll not quite be up for your usual long hard Wednesday endurance ride. If you continue training unabated, burnout may be on its way.

Avoiding Burnout

It's not always easy to figure out how hard you can push, until you push yourself too far. Avoiding burnout takes some experience.

What you can and cannot do also depends upon how other specific stresses may affect you. For example, I get travel sick easily. I can go out of town to race a couple of weekends in a row. Any more than that and I turn green and yellow and become reasonably worthless on a bike. To avoid travel burnout, I don't travel in the weeks before I've got a big race planned.

The way in which you might change your workouts when you're over-stressed from cycling is aided by understanding some exercise physiology: Speed and aerobic and anaerobic fitness start declining in as little as 3 or 4 days. Endurance and strength can be maintained with endurance rides or strength workouts every 1 to 2 weeks.

If you normally incorporate a couple of endurance or long rides a week, and you start getting tired of riding, you can safely sacrifice one of these long rides to give yourself a physical or mental break.

If you normally include 10 sprints in your Tuesday workouts, you'd be better off doing 5 sprints on Tuesday at your usual all-out sprint pace, rather than the full 10 at less than total anaerobic effort.

Summary

- Burnout happens to us all.
- Be flexible in modifying your schedule if necessary.
- Trim miles and mental fatigue by reducing endurance rides first.
- Cut back on distance and repeats when tired, but not max effort.
- Find something else to do—mountain bike, tour, run, go surfing.
- It's okay to take a day or two off.

CHAPTER 22

How Much Is Enough?

As I was driving out to Borrego for a time trial, I heard a radio program on NPR. The show was entitled "How Much Is Enough?" The question was: "How much money is enough?" Someone is always making more, having more. How much is enough? If you spend all your time making money, when will you enjoy it?

A millionaire interviewed needed more.

A family of five, with an annual income of $30,000, was quite happy. The husband worked outside the home and earned the $30,000. The wife worked in the home, spending time with the kids, recycling things, clipping discount coupons. They felt they had plenty.

A man worked from 1970 to 1977, saved $70,000, retired on the interest, hadn't worked a day since, and felt $5,000 a year was plenty.

How much bicycling is enough, and how good is good enough? Is a 30-minute 10-mile time trial good enough? Do you need to go 27 minutes? 25? 23? 21?

Winning interviewed Robert Millar, who came to the conclusion that even if he didn't win the Tour's mountains jersey, or place in the top 10 in the GC, it was enough that he was still riding—but he didn't always feel that way. He had felt he had to win the Tour at one time in his life.

What Is a Champion?

With every first-place champion, there are those who did not place first. Are they any less champions? Why do we ride, train, race?

A club member, a first-time Nationals competitor, told me she was motivated to train even harder and improve her time-trial performance next year. She thought of herself as mediocre because her time was slow compared to the first-place champion's.

A club member, a first-place champion, was disappointed because the winning time was slower than a champion from a different age group. Several former national champions who "only placed" were bitterly disappointed. A national champion who didn't quite manage to place was devastated.

Why are we so hard on ourselves?

A top-10 rider rode for all he was worth, at a heart rate of 175, for almost an hour. It is true others were faster—that's the reality—but he worked as hard as he could. He is just as much a champion.

George Sheehan used to be a front-runner, in contention for winning the running races he entered. As he got older, he found himself farther and farther back in the pack. Soon he was at the rear of races. What George found, to his surprise, was that those at the back of the pack were not lollygagging and chatting as he had assumed. They were working just as hard!

Others Think You're Great

How many of you think you are not that great, because there are others in the club stronger than you are? Your co-workers, friends, and others ask you naive questions, such as "When are you going to Europe to ride the Tour de France?"

They think that since you ride 100 miles per week (or is that 200, or 300?) you are the fittest of the species. They think that because you wear that club jersey and go out and ride you must be a fantastic rider.

They just don't understand, do they? You think that because you can barely keep up with the B ride, or the A ride, or the Sandtrap ride, or racing Cat 4, or Cat 3 or Cat 2, or masters locally, or nationally, or internationally, or barely medal, that you are not good enough. But how much is enough? Maybe you're wrong. Maybe your co-workers and friends are right. You are great. Riding is great. Roll in it. Immerse yourself. Exalt. You are having the ride of your life!

CHAPTER 23

Confidence

Almost every coach and athlete feels that self-confidence is vital to successful athletic competition. Where does confidence arise? How can it be nurtured?

What We're Talking About

Confidence is the realistic expectation of success or of achieving one's goals. It's what athletes reasonably hope to do, not what they dream of achieving.

Confident athletes are prepared. Confident athletes accurately judge their abilities and have appropriate goals.

Confidence about future performance is based upon past performance. Confidence is an expression of one's perceived self-worth. Confidence in sport is related to past experiences within and outside of sport.

An important characteristic of the confident is the belief in their ability to become competent.

Overconfidence

Overconfidence is a false confidence that looks beyond one's true ability.

Sometimes overconfidence comes from athletes who are honestly lacking in a realistic appraisal of their abilities. Sometimes overconfidence comes from coaches or parents who unrealistically inflate and pamper an athlete. Since this overconfidence is not based on reality, failure and disappointment are likely results.

False confidence is also seen in athletes who lack confidence but make a display of acting confident and misrepresent their abilities to others. Such athletes may hope for a lucky break in a race. Often others perceive the hoax more readily than does the athlete.

This behavior makes it more difficult for the athlete to psychologically reconcile poor performance with inflated claims. In this psychological fraud, the perpetrator is often the victim.

Such athletes avoid situations threatening their confidence. They fake injury and mechanical problems. They find it difficult to admit errors and do not accept responsibility for their errors. They find excuses. Out of fear of failure, they avoid situations where they might challenge themselves and improve.

Sometimes false confidence arises from coaches and others whose credos include "Think positive," "You can achieve any goal you set your sights on," "You must believe you should win every time, or you are a loser."

Positive thinking alone does not give confidence. Confidence must be earned, not stolen from false hope.

Underconfidence

A lack of confidence, underconfidence or diffidence, reflects a lower expectation of success than might be reasonably achieved based on the athlete's abilities.

Underconfident athletes focus on their shortcomings rather than on their strengths. Underconfident athletes are tentative and suffer from anxiety, loss of concentration, and uncertainty of purpose. Fear of failure is also present.

Mistakes, errors, and poor performances that occur in all athletes reinforce the lack of confidence in the underconfident athlete. In contrast, the self-confident athlete accepts poor results and learns, adapts, and improves as a result of those experiences.

Self-Fulfilling Prophecies

Confronted with a range of potential performance based on ability, the confident athlete strives toward the higher end of the range. The underconfident athlete is drawn to the lower end.

Although unreasonably high expectations may lead to disappointment, reasonably high expectations of performance do draw athletes to those higher levels and result in positive self-fulfilling prophecies.

Self-doubt and expectations of failure often lead to negative self-fulfilling prophecies and confirm negative self-images.

Confidence Examples

A new rider considered entering a 10-mile time trial. She was concerned that she might fall down while being held for the start. To gain the confidence to enter the race, she practiced starts with her boyfriend.

Another new rider wanted to be national champion his second year of racing. He set himself up to win at all costs. When he failed in his attempt, he gave up bike racing.

A racer, uncertain of his competition, timidly rode the back of a three-up track sprint. His timidity lost him the race. Later, through consolation rounds, he again faced the same opponents. Told that other riders he had previously outsprinted could beat these same two opponents, he became more confident and aggressive, and outsprinted these same two opponents.

How to Get Confidence

- Set realistic, specific, short- and long-term goals.
- Train to achieve goals incrementally and progressively.
- Improve the performance components of your sport, including fitness, tactics, and techniques.
- Familiarize yourself with pre-event, event, and post-event routines and strategies.
- Think positively, in realistic terms.
- Experience success.
- After a poor performance, learn, correct, and adapt.
- Improve performance.

CHAPTER 24

Visualization

We've heard a little bit about this subject. Few of us practice it with regularity or train this way. There are rumors that the Russians and other Eastern Block countries spend as much as one-third of their training time with visualization techniques.

Visualize Success

You want to "see in your mind's eye" the action you wish to accomplish, and you want to see yourself being successful.

One of the first books I read on visualization was a story about a coach who had used visualization with a basketball team. He had his athletes spend one-quarter of their training time visualizing themselves throwing basketballs at hoops, rather than actually practicing on the court. At the end of the season the team did much worse than expected. It turned out the athletes were seeing themselves throwing shots at the basket but saw themselves missing!

Let Negative Images Float Away

Sometimes when thinking about an action, you'll find other thoughts—either stray thoughts or negative images—appear in your consciousness. The easiest way to deal with these images is to let them drift away. Don't focus on them, don't dwell on them. See the images grow smaller and dimmer, and drift away; or just return to the desired image.

Enhance Positive Images

You can change the images you see. If you picture yourself on a bicycle, you can change the size of the image. You can focus on certain parts of the image—for example, your legs. You can make those characteristics you wish to enhance larger, stronger, bolder, brighter. You can visualize other elements as well. You can call up sounds, pressure/touch sensations, smell.

Focus on Your Objectives

Here's a little something to try when riding your bike. Ride along and find a pothole. Try not to ride in the pothole while looking steadfastly at the pothole.

Now try again, this time looking away from the pothole and focusing on something else. It is almost always easier to avoid the pothole by not looking at it. Look away from negative images.

I am not saying that negative thoughts and images don't exist—just focus your attention elsewhere or you may drift toward those negative images.

Making a tight corner in a time trial, or a crit? Don't look at the curb. Don't look at that gravel. Look inside the curb, look beyond the corner. Look where you want to go. It's easy to make that turnaround. It's easy to make that corner.

Augment Images with Sound

Want to improve your track starts? Need to get up to speed more quickly for the kilo? Vic Copeland taught me, when starting from a standstill and getting up to speed, to say "POW! POW! POW!" with each push down on the pedal stroke.

When you think something, that process occurs in just one side of your brain. When you say something aloud, both sides of your brain hear and act on that information.

Try These Experiments

Try this on your stationary trainer: Get so that you are working hard during isolated leg training. Let your mind drift—watch someone else, think about what one of your friends said earlier, or chat with someone nearby. Look at your cadence.

Now focus on your leg. Either look at your leg directly, or close your eyes and picture it as you pedal. Say to yourself "PUSH! PUSH! PUSH!" with each pedal stroke, and really push! Look again at your cadence. It is possible to get that cadence higher and do more work, isn't it?

Leaving home and feel you've forgotten something you need for the Thursday stationary trainer class? Close your eyes a minute. See a picture of yourself on the bike. See that image. Now look at the parts of that image. Enumerate the parts. Trainer, bike, shoes, bike shorts, etc. You may see and remember that forgotten item!

Climbing about the same pace as a rider 100 meters ahead of you on a climb? Working hard? Look at that rider. Focus on that rider. See a string coming from the back of that rider. See the string coming to you. See yourself pulling that string, reeling in that rider closer and closer. Sometimes it's baffling how much faster you can ride!

Did you try a spin workout in class and get up to 115 rpm? Go back to your house and try to replicate the Thursday workouts? Sometimes you can. Sometimes you can't get your spin or your heart rate nearly as high? Of course you can! But when the motivation is different, when you really don't believe you will see those numbers on your computer, it makes it harder for them to appear.

Spinning and finding it hard to maintain 110 rpm? Close your eyes. Count to 10 while pushing down on your left foot, pulling up on your right. Now switch, count to 11 while pushing with your right, pulling with your left. Now switch, count to 12 while pushing with your left, pulling with your right. Keep changing back and forth while building a pyramid to 20 strokes while concentrating on pushing/pulling, then let the pyramid decrease—20, 19, 18, down to 10 again. I find it easier to keep spinning this way. Not only that, it takes a full 3 minutes to do this pyramid at 110 rpm.

Be Alert for Visualization Tricks

There are many tricks that will allow you to focus on the task at hand, make the task easier, and get a better workout that's more fun at the same time. Be alert for these tricks, ask others about tricks, make them up on your own!

CHAPTER 25

The Optimist's Creed

Promise yourself:

- To be so strong that nothing can disturb your peace of mind.
- To talk health, happiness, and prosperity to every person you meet.
- To make all of your friends feel there is something in them.
- To look at the sunny side of everything and make your optimism come true.
- To think of the best, to work only for the best, and to expect only the best.
- To be just as enthusiastic about the success of others as you are about your own.
- To forget the mistakes of the past and press on to the greater achievements of the future.
- To wear a cheerful countenance at all times and give every living creature you meet a smile.
- To give so much time to the improvement of yourself that you have no time to criticize others.
- To be too large for worry, too noble for anger, too strong for fear, and too happy to permit the presence of trouble.

Appendix A: Training Logs

Training Logs Explained

Charting your workouts and results is an important part of training. Monitoring your progress allows you to evaluate your efforts and performance. This allows you to modify your future training if necessary. Review of past performance allows you to understand your present condition and anticipate the future. Blank logs are found on pages 247 and 249.

MONTHLY TRAINING LOG

The monthly training log records, on a single page, an overview of the month's training. It gives only the general flavor of a workout. A single line records the basic information of the workout.

Distance traveled, or time spent, is the most basic measure of an workout—its duration. The group ridden with, the type of workout, the location, and the intensity gives some detail to the day. Other information of interest or short details can be given on the single line. Morning pulse or weight may be recorded.

The form is simple. More complex training diaries and computerized record systems are available, but if they take too much time you might not use them. Copy this log and use it. As you develop your own specific requirements, modify it to suit your needs.

Figure A-1 Monthly Training Log

Date	Dist	Group	Type	Location	Intensity	Particulars	Pulse	Weight
1								
2								
3								
4								
5								
6								
7								
8								
9								
10								
11								
12								
13								
14								
15								
16								
17								
18								
19								
20								
21								
22								
23								
24								
25								
26								
27								
28								
29								
30								
31								
Total								
PR's								

SPECIFIC WORKOUT LOG

This workout log is used to record details of a workout. Use the specific workout log when certain details about the workout will prove helpful for future training or goal setting. Most group and social rides are not recorded in this format. Record specific details of a workout when you perform a specific road or trainer workout.

Record the day of the week and the date on the top of the workout. The general format or type of workout is recorded next. For example: time trial, intervals, sprints, or leg speed workout.

Each of the following lines can be used to record details of each exercise within the workout. Succeeding columns might record the duration, type, gear, cadence, and position. The bottom boxes are used to record heart rates at the end of hard efforts and recovery heart rates for 30-second intervals up to two minutes thereafter.

Figure A–2 **Specific Workout Log Example**

Day: Thursday   **Date:** Jan 6, 199X
Format: Introduction to Spinning
         Isolated Leg Training

15 min	Warm-up	42/17	to 100 rpm	Hoods
8′	Spin	42/17	to 110	Drops
7′	Spin	42/17	to 120	Drops
1′	ILT	42/15	40+	Tops
160 bpm	148	127	118	106

Figure A–3 **Specific Workout Log**

Day: **Date:**
Format:

Day: **Date:**
Format:

Day: **Date:**
Format:

Day: **Date:**
Format:

Day: **Date:**
Format:

Day: **Date:**
Format:

Weight-Training Log Explained

Recording your weight-training workouts is important. Weight training often involves lifting as much weight as possible for a specified number of repetitions. Records allow you to know exactly how much weight to lift in subsequent workouts.

WHY KEEP A WEIGHT-TRAINING LOG?

Lifting weights can be hard work. The differences between sessions and the gains you make are great initially and then modest.

A record of your past workouts lets you know at what level you expect to perform your next workout. When you know that you have performed 12 repetitions last session and you are feeling strong, you know to expect to lift more weight or perform more repetitions in your current workout.

Records from previous years can help you determine suitable weight-training goals for this year.

The chart I have developed records one month's activity. Modify it depending upon the exercises you perform. A full month's blank chart follows the sample below. Here's how I fill it out:

Date	CU	PU	BE	Sit	Jp	StepUp	Squats	More
						2 2 3		
1						] | |	] | |	
2						] | |	] | |	
3						] | |	] | |	
4						] | |	] | |	
5						] | |	] | |	

- I write the month and year in the first column, under Date.
- I use abbreviations for the exercises I use. For example:

  CU is chin-ups.
  PU is push-ups.
  BE is back extensions.
  Sit is sit-ups.
  Jp is jumps.

- Some exercises I perform only once in a session. Sometimes I perform several sets in a session. I use a bracket and lines to separate my recording box into sections:] | |
- Step-ups are my favorite exercise. I usually perform 2 sets of 2 steps, or 16 inches, and a third set of 3 steps or 24 inches.

- x] a | b | c |
- x is the weight that I am using.
- a, b, and c are the number of reps performed for each of three sets.

Figure A–5 **Weight-Training Log**

Date	CU	PU	Sit	Jp	StepUp	Lg Pull	Squats
					1 2 3		
1					] | |	] | |	] | |
2					] | |	] | |	] | |
3					] | |	] | |	] | |
4					] | |	] | |	] | |
5					] | |	] | |	] | |
6					] | |	] | |	] | |
7					] | |	] | |	] | |
8					] | |	] | |	] | |
9					] | |	] | |	] | |
10					] | |	] | |	] | |
11					] | |	] | |	] | |
12					] | |	] | |	] | |
13					] | |	] | |	] | |
14					] | |	] | |	] | |
15					] | |	] | |	] | |
16					] | |	] | |	] | |
17					] | |	] | |	] | |
18					] | |	] | |	] | |
19					] | |	] | |	] | |
20					] | |	] | |	] | |
21					] | |	] | |	] | |
22					] | |	] | |	] | |
23					] | |	] | |	] | |
24					] | |	] | |	] | |
25					] | |	] | |	] | |
26					] | |	] | |	] | |
27					] | |	] | |	] | |
28					] | |	] | |	] | |
29					] | |	] | |	] | |
30					] | |	] | |	] | |
31					] | |	] | |	] | |

LgPress	LgExt	ToeRs	LgCurls	SShrugs	TriCurls	BBCurls
] | |	] | |	] | |	] | |	] | |	] | |	] | |
] | |	] | |	] | |	] | |	] | |	] | |	] | |
] | |	] | |	] | |	] | |	] | |	] | |	] | |
] | |	] | |	] | |	] | |	] | |	] | |	] | |
] | |	] | |	] | |	] | |	] | |	] | |	] | |
] | |	] | |	] | |	] | |	] | |	] | |	] | |
] | |	] | |	] | |	] | |	] | |	] | |	] | |
] | |	] | |	] | |	] | |	] | |	] | |	] | |
] | |	] | |	] | |	] | |	] | |	] | |	] | |
] | |	] | |	] | |	] | |	] | |	] | |	] | |
] | |	] | |	] | |	] | |	] | |	] | |	] | |
] | |	] | |	] | |	] | |	] | |	] | |	] | |
] | |	] | |	] | |	] | |	] | |	] | |	] | |
] | |	] | |	] | |	] | |	] | |	] | |	] | |
] | |	] | |	] | |	] | |	] | |	] | |	] | |
] | |	] | |	] | |	] | |	] | |	] | |	] | |
] | |	] | |	] | |	] | |	] | |	] | |	] | |
] | |	] | |	] | |	] | |	] | |	] | |	] | |
] | |	] | |	] | |	] | |	] | |	] | |	] | |
] | |	] | |	] | |	] | |	] | |	] | |	] | |
] | |	] | |	] | |	] | |	] | |	] | |	] | |
] | |	] | |	] | |	] | |	] | |	] | |	] | |
] | |	] | |	] | |	] | |	] | |	] | |	] | |
] | |	] | |	] | |	] | |	] | |	] | |	] | |
] | |	] | |	] | |	] | |	] | |	] | |	] | |
] | |	] | |	] | |	] | |	] | |	] | |	] | |
] | |	] | |	] | |	] | |	] | |	] | |	] | |
] | |	] | |	] | |	] | |	] | |	] | |	] | |

Appendix B: Health and Medical

Road Rash

This most common of bicycling injuries can be treated in different ways. The right way reduces healing time and scarring and allows you to return to your bike promptly.

PREVENTION

Learn bike-handling skills to help prevent falling. Ride defensively, especially in traffic and around squirrelly riders. Always wear a helmet.

TREATMENT OBJECTIVES

The objective of treatment is to heal the tissues as rapidly and effectively as possible. Goals of therapy include preventing further damage to the skin and not allowing the depth of the rash to increase in severity.

What can go wrong? The rash can heal with scarring. The rash can take longer to heal than needed—because of infection, for example. Or the rash can heal OK but be more painful than necessary during the healing process.

GRADING ROAD RASH

Severity of road rash is similar to that of burns. Rash can be:

- First degree: Only the surface is reddened. This problem does not require active treatment.
- Second degree: The surface layer of the skin is broken, but a deep layer remains that will allow the skin to replace itself and heal without significant scarring.
- Third degree: The skin is entirely removed, perhaps with underlying layers of fat and other supporting tissue structures exposed. Such damage may require skin grafting and is beyond the scope of this book. Seek immediate medical attention.

OLD-STYLE TREATMENT

There are two general methods of treatment for second-degree road rash. The first is the traditional "let nature take its course" approach, which is also called the "open method." This involves cleaning the wound with soap and water, hydrogen peroxide, and iodide or something similar, and then allowing the wound to dry out, form a scab, and "heal on its own."

This method does have its drawbacks for all but the most superficial and small road rashes. Just because you clean it once doesn't mean it won't get infected. Bacteria thrive on damaged skin. Infection can deepen the depth of the rash, meaning that scarring and delayed healing is more likely. Scabs can crack and become painful. Scabbed areas don't receive oxygen well from the surrounding air and so take much longer to heal.

MODERN THINKING

The alternative is the "closed approach"—frequent cleansings and the application of topical antibiotics and dressings that keep the road rash moist and closed to the air. The area is cleansed at least daily with wet compresses or bathing. Superficial debris is gently removed. An effort is made to remove soft-forming exudates (the beginnings of scabs) with gentle scrubbing. Pink, healthy, new-forming skin is what you want to see.

MODERN-THINKING SUPPLIES

Polysporin, silver sulfadiazine (Silvadene), or mupirocin (Bactroban) is applied. A Vaseline gauze (Adaptic) is placed over this. This is a non-stick mesh that allows removal of the dressing without sticking. Padding in the form of gauze squares may be applied. Then, a conforming gauze roll is wrapped around the area and taped in place. Finally, a tube stretch gauze (Tubigauze) is applied over this to keep everything in place and tidy.

Alternatively, Tegaderm (3M) or Bioclusive (Johnson & Johnson) alone may be stretched over the antibiotic.

The result is a dressing that allows maximum protection of the wound, minimum risk of infection, prevention of scabbing and its attendant cracking and pain, and healing as fast as possible.

SIDE EFFECTS

Those persons allergic to sulfa drugs should avoid sulfadiazine. Mupirocin is a little better at controlling skin infections, but it's more expensive. Polysporin—available over-the-counter—is much less likely to irritate the skin than Neosporin.

WATCH FOR SUNBURN ON ROAD RASH

As the skin nears complete healing, you may be tempted to allow your technique to become lax. Sun exposure may cause the skin to remain permanently darkened after healing. Be sure to keep your rash covered until completely healed. Use adequate (SPF>18) sunscreen.

Saddle Sores

Sores of the butt are a common occupational hazard for the bicycle rider. Many causes can be avoided. Specific treatment is available if saddle sores do develop.

WHAT WE'RE TALKING ABOUT

The phrase saddle sores is used by different riders to refer to a number of separate problems involving the skin of the upper thigh and of the rear end. Pressure, friction, and infection are the three main causes of saddle sores.

Furuncles and Folliculitis

Blocked and/or infected glands and lumps are a common cycling problem. These painful bumps are classic saddle sores.

Ischial Tuberosity Pain

This is pain in the area of the pelvic bones that bear your weight on the bicycle seat. The ischial tuberosities are the "sitting bones." Occasionally, pain in this area progresses to either a local bursitis or ulceration.

Chafing of the Thigh

Chafing of the inside of the upper leg is common among cyclists. It occurs because of friction caused by the repeated rubbing of the inside thigh during the up and down motion of the pedal stroke.

Many cyclists note that the inside of their shorts pill and wear with friction. When this happens to your inner thighs, redness and discomfort are the results. Dampness of the cycling short related to sweat production and the lack of breathability of the short's material may make the problem worse.

Skin Ulceration

Skin that is missing its topmost surface layers and is denuded is ulcerated. This is sometimes an extreme result of rubbing or pressure.

Relatively Rare Problems

Subcutaneous nodules: These are a specific type of lump found in elite male cyclists near the scrotum, sometimes called "extra testicles."

Tailbone abscess: A genetic predisposition to a blocked pilonidal sinus may be aggravated by cycling and become infected. Surgical treatment is often advised.

SADDLE SORE THEORY

Classic saddle sores have two prevalent theories behind their origin.

The first has to do with blocked glands and infection. Therefore, treatment is directed at preventing pore blockage and reducing the level of skin bacteria. This is old-school thinking.

Modern theory has to do with saddle pressure. According to this theory, increased saddle pressure (which often arises through increased miles) prevents small blood vessels from bringing blood to the skin and the skin gets less nutrients. This causes a breakdown in the skin's defenses and a saddle sore develops.

PREVENTION

- Keep yourself dry. Modern synthetics wick away moisture and are softer on the skin than traditional leather chamois. Don't continue to wear sweat-drenched shorts after riding. Change into loose shorts that allow air to circulate. After bathing, allow your crotch to dry completely before putting on tight-fitting shorts or cycling shorts. Powder in your shorts can help to prevent chafing that may lead to irritation and infected blocked glands.
- Keep yourself clean.
- Wear synthetic, padded cycling shorts.
- Always wear clean cycling shorts. Avoid wearing the same shorts two days in a row without laundering. Soiled shorts not only have more bacteria, they don't breathe as well as freshly laundered ones.
- Avoid cycling shorts with seams in areas that either rub the inside thigh or upon which pressure is placed.
- Do not suddenly and drastically increase your weekly mileage.
- Use seats that provide enough padding or support and spread the support over as wide an area as is compatible with your anatomy.
- Check your seat position.
- Avoid shaving above the short line to the groin. This often results in "red spots," caused by irritation and infection.

SELF-TREATMENT

- Apply all the preventative measures described above.
- Modify your training. You don't have to stop cycling but you may need to back off. This is not the time to increase mileage. A couple of years ago when I had some bad saddle sores, I modified my routine. Tuesday was hill sprints, Wednesday long hill climbing, and Thursday hill intervals—all done out of the saddle and off my sores!
- Soak in a comfortably hot bath three times a day for 15 minutes to allow

boils to come to the surface and drain. Hot-water soaks increase blood circulation to the inflamed area, allowing more of the body's healing factors access to the area.

- For classic saddle sores or ischial-tuberosity pain, pad your skin with padded tape or moleskin. You may want to reduce the tackiness of moleskin by first applying it to something other than your skin. Leave some tack so that it will still stick, but not so much that it pulls off your skin and hair when you remove it later.
- Another possibility is to take a couple of Band-Aids or a layer of moleskin and cut out a small hole to accommodate the sore—effectively padding around the sore and taking pressure off the sore itself.
- The extra padding of a second pair of shorts worn over the first may help.
- A padded seat cover may help.
- A different seat may help.
- Suspension may help. Rear-end suspension or beamed seat tubes reduce saddle pressure.
- A modification of seat position—nose up or down, forward or back, up or down—may help.
- Friction-related problems may be helped by an emollient, such as Vaseline.
- Topical cortisone creams are used by some, but have never been proven to be of benefit.

MEDICAL AND SURGICAL TREATMENT
- If the area around the sore is infected, it may require surgical drainage or antibiotics.
- Uninfected sores that remain painful, swollen, hard lumps can occasionally be treated with a cortisone injection.
- Occasionally surgery may be required to removed chronic cysts.

Crotchitis

Crotchitis is irritation or inflammation of the crotch. Redness, itching, and pain are problems in this area. Crotchitis is common in women—specifically irritation of the skin around the vagina, the clitoris, and the urethra. Crotchitis is distinctive from saddle sores, discussed above.

PREVENTION

The best treatment is prevention. Some general measures will help almost all cases of crotchitis. Some treatments may improve some causes of crotchitis but actually may make other cases worse! It is therefore important to determine the cause of your crotchitis.

CAUSES OF CROTCHITIS

Many cases of crotchitis are related to a combination of factors.

- Warmth
- Moisture
- Hygiene and irritants
- Friction
- Bicycle position and saddle
- Medical problems, including dermatitis
- Allergy
- Vaginal infections

Warmth and Moisture

Warmth and moisture aggravate most cases of crotchitis. Avoid traveling to races or rides in your car already wearing your bike shorts. Change into bike shorts when you arrive. Use bike shorts with a breathable, moisture-wicking crotch. Change out of moist or wet bicycling shorts as soon as you can after riding. Wear loose-fitting shorts or a skirt. Avoid tight-fitting non-breathing underwear or wear no underwear.

Allow ventilation to cool and dry the area. Moisture and warmth causes yeast overgrowth—"jock crotch." Antifungal powders, found in athlete's foot products, may help reduce yeast overgrowth. Over-the-counter cortisone cream may also reduce irritation.

Hygiene and Irritants

Stool is a powerful irritant. Clean yourself properly. Overzealous hygiene can be just as much of a problem as a lack of hygiene. When you are irritated, wiping and rubbing can cause chafing and further irritation. Since the anus always has some bacteria and since irritated skin is prone to worsen and get infected, overzealous wiping must be avoided. Avoid wiping affected areas with rough toilet tissue.

Wipe from front to back. Don't carry bacteria toward your vagina and urethra. Not only is crotchitis worsened, but urinary tract infections and vaginal infections may result as well.

Avoid local irritants such as harsh soaps.

If crotchitis extends to areas you need to wipe to keep clean, consider using a facial tissue, gentle, medicated over-the-counter products such as Tucks, or plain water. Clean and then pat—not wipe—dry.

Friction

Friction can be minimized by using an emollient skin preparation, such as Vaseline. A seat pad or cover fitted over your saddle may allow slight movement and function similarly to a sock in your shoe.

Wearing two pairs of lightweight bicycling shorts or a lightweight bicycling liner may help to reduce friction-caused crotchitis. But if crotchitis is related to warmth and moisture, doubling up on your shorts may make things worse.

Bicycle Position

Most bicycles are sold for men, and the top tube stem length results in too much reach for most women. This puts extra pressure on the crotch. Make sure your bicycle position is not too stretched out.

Saddle

Saddle position and saddle type may be factors relating to crotchitis. Consider seat angle. Nose down slightly may help, especially for time-trial events or crits where you are in an aerodynamic position and putting a lot of pressure on the crotch. Some women prefer a nose-up position so that the saddle presses more on the pubic bone and less on the soft tissues around the vagina.

Move around frequently—get off that saddle when you can. Stand up on your pedals to relieve crotch friction and pressure. Climb hills standing up periodically. When descending, put weight on your pedals and get off your saddle. This allows moving air to cool and dry your crotch while you relieve pressure. If riding tandem, be sure to take frequent crotch breaks by getting out of the saddle at stop signs and stop lights and by standing with your partner at least every 15 minutes.

Terry saddles have padding and are less stiff. Many women report that although they feel no different from other saddles while riding, at the end of a ride their crotches don't hurt as much. Semi-terminal cases of crotchitis may require drastic measures—cutting or paring your seat may be necessary to keep riding.

Medical Problems

Riders with skin conditions such as psoriasis or excema may have flare-ups in this area related to friction and other general factors listed above. Prescription strength cortisone creams are often the best help for this.

Allergies

Many riders use a wide variety of products in this area that may cause allergies. To help with saddle sores near the crotch, riders may use tapes or pads to which they may have a tape allergy. This worsens saddle sores into saddle sores plus crotchitis!

Some riders use perfumed or chemically treated products, including sprays, sanitary napkins, or lubricating oils to which they may be allergic. These can cause or worsen crotchitis.

Vaginal Infections

The extra moisture related to a vaginal infection may worsen crotchitis. Treating the underlying vaginal discharge may help improve crotchitis. Infected or otherwise blocked sweat or other glands may develop into crotchitis if friction worsens these conditions.

Why Am I Tired?

Riders may find themselves tired and wonder why. Probably your tiredness falls into one of these categories:

- Stress, emotional turmoil
- Inadequate sleep
- Overtraining/burnout
- Increased load too quickly
- Too rapid weight loss
- Inadequate nutrition
- Medical problems

Stress

Stress is one of the most common reasons why athletes and nonathletes alike are tired. Most people think of stress as bad events in their lives. Actually, stress is change.

Good changes and bad changes are stressful. Getting a new bicycle and figuring out all the components you want to put on it and being excited about it may be good, but your increased anxiety may cause you to lose sleep and get exhausted just in planning, never mind riding, your new bike! Marriages, separations, deaths in the family, job changes, new purchases, and accidents are some of the big stresses in our lives. Get too many of them in a year and most of us become tired, perhaps as a way of avoiding these stressful situations.

Consider the important people and things in your life: family and friends, job, money, lover(s). Have these changed recently? If so, stress may contribute to your fatigue.

Inadequate Sleep

Sleep loss is an understandable cause of fatigue. Inadequate sleep is often related to stresses already discussed. By going to sleep at a regular hour and arising at a regular hour, you set the pattern for good sleep habits. Quiet activity 15 minutes before sleep—reading a book or listening to soft music—may also help you sleep better.

Burnout, Overtraining

We hear the terms. What do they mean? Again, they may be psychological or physical defense mechanisms for dealing with too much at once.

Think of burnout as a psychological or emotional situation, overtraining as a physical one. They are often intertwined. We are just beginning to understand the neurohormonal basis of fatigue.

You may be enthusiastic about getting stronger and read a program on interval training. If you begin a serious program of interval training, even with a good base, it is difficult to maintain such a program without diversity and measurable results or other positive feedback. It's easy to suffer mental burnout. If you do the same workouts day in day out, even though they may be physiologically sound, it's easy to suffer burnout.

My rule of thumb is, "When you look at the bike in the morning, are you raring to get on it or do you groan inside about the workout you have set for yourself?" You know what the latter means!

If you are working hard on the bike without proper recovery, you may become tired because of overtraining.

Push, yes, but not too hard all the time. You need some easy days, some quiet, friendly rides, maybe some bike touring. Ignore recovery training and you may dig yourself a hole that not even a week or two off the bike can cure—then you may really lose fitness!

If you go from 100 to 200 miles in a couple of weeks, you may be mentally eager to ride more, but your body may say: No! It is important to have a measured increase in workload to avoid fatigue. If you increase your mileage more than 10% per week, you should cut back on intensity or you're likely to be tired!

Too Much Weight Loss

Many athletes rightly try to lose weight to improve their performance. Weight loss of more than one to two pounds weekly, though, often results in fatigue and worsens performance.

Inadequate Nutrition

Your body needs calories, nutrients, and fluids to work properly. If you ride more than a couple of hours and get tired, the problem may be simply that you need to eat and drink more!

Medical Causes

Medical causes are the least frequent explanation for fatigue. Nonetheless, if your fatigue lasts more than a month or two, a medical checkup may be wise.

Some causes include anemia, diabetes, low thyroid function, or other organ disease of almost any kind; infectious diseases; or depression.

I remember a runner from San Diego State coming to see me when I was first in practice. He was complaining of tiredness and said his coach told him to have a medical checkup. He felt he should be running faster. I asked him what his 10K time was and he said 32 minutes. Right, I said to myself, I should be as tired as this guy.

Well, I ran the usual tests. I learned something from that runner. His thyroid test showed a level of extreme under-activity, a level I had almost never seen before. When I replaced his thyroid hormone, his 10K time dropped to 29 something and he won a national title.

Chronic fatigue syndrome is a poorly understood medical condition. No consistent physical findings, laboratory tests, causes, or treatments exist. As is the case with other medical problems that remain poorly defined, personal testimonial and anecdotal reports, often with considerable conviction, cloud scientific evidence. At one time, the Epstein-Barr virus was thought to be related to this problem. Current evidence dismisses this possibility. It is clear that depression is often present.

Medical causes for fatigue are unusual, but when one is found, help may be dramatic.

Glossary

Aerobic With oxygen as a fuel source. Implied intensity is below anaerobic level. Implied level of work is low enough that buildup of lactic acid is avoided and exercise can be continued for prolonged periods.

Aerodynamic With reduced air resistance.

Anaerobic Without the presence of oxygen. Implies a high level of work intensity that can only be maintained for relatively short periods of time. A very short energy production system—that of creatine phosphate—can supply energy need for about 10 seconds without the production of lactic acid. Other anaerobic efforts result in higher levels of lactic acid.

ATP Adenosine triphosphate. A chemical in cells serving as an immediate source of energy.

Attack An aggressive high-speed jump away from other riders.

Block To impede the progress of the pack in order. Normally for tactical reasons, when a teammate is in a break.

Blow Up Go out too fast and not be able to continue.

Bonk Run out of energy, tire.

Break One or more riders forming a small group ahead of the main pack.

Bridge To join a rider or group of riders ahead. Bridging usually implies a tactical effort in which only a rider or small group reaches the group ahead. If the whole pack rejoins, it is not a bridge. The group ahead was merely caught.

Cadence Revolutions per minute of pedal stroke.

Cardiovascular Referring to the heart and blood vessels.

Chase   To try to catch a rider or group ahead.

Circuit Race   Multi-lap road-race event on courses more than one mile.

Clincher   Bicycle tire with a bead holding it onto the rim. A separate tube within holds air.

Creatine Phosphate   A chemical in cells that can briefly replenish ATP and thereby produce energy for very short (up to 10 seconds) events.

Criterium   Multi-lap road race in which the distance of each lap is one mile or less.

Derailleur   Gear-shifting mechanism on a bicycle.

Disc Wheel   Solid wheel used for its aerodynamic advantage.

Domestique   Team worker sacrificing his chances for that of a teammate.

Drafting   Riding behind others in their slipstream.

Drop   Ride faster and away from another rider or group.

Drops   The lower part of down-turned handlebars.

Duration   Length of time spent performing an interval. If work is continuous, volume and duration are the same.

Echelon   Staggered riders drafting in a crosswind.

Endurance   Ability to last.

Energy   The capacity to perform work.

Ergogenic   Special substances or treatments used to improve physiological, psychological, or biomechanical function. They may include nutritional, pharmacological, or psychological approaches.

Fartlek   "Speed play," unstructured intervals.

Fatigue   The inability to maintain a level of work.

Feed Zone   Designated area along a road race where racers may be handed up food and drink from the roadside.

Field   The main group of riders, pack, peloton.

Field Sprint   Sprint of the main pack for the finish line.

Flexibility   The range of motion of the body's joints.

Flyer   Attack and effort off the front, often solo.

Force the Pace   Go harder and increase the pace of the group.

Fred   Novice rider, or one who rides that way.

Gap   Distance between individuals or groups.

G.C.   General Classification. Overall placing in a stage race.

Glucose   A simple sugar. Used for energy by the body.

Glycogen   A complex sugar. A form of storage energy in the body.

Hammer   Hard, sustained effort.

Hang On   To just manage to stay with the pack.

Hoods   The covers of the brake handles where riders frequently rest their hands.

Hook   To rub one's back wheel against the front of another rider. The rider behind, whose front wheel is rubbed, frequently crashes. Sometimes inadvertent, sometimes an illegal aggressive racing tactic.

Intensity   Load or speed of work.

Interval   Riding hard for relatively short periods.

Isolated Leg Training (ILT)   Training technique of riding with one leg to improve performance.

Jam   High-speed riding.

Jump   A short, quick burst of speed.

Kick   Final burst of speed.

Lactic Acid   A product of the body's metabolism. Normally the blood contains less than one millimole of lactic acid per liter. Efforts up to the anaerobic threshold may result in levels of up to four millimoles per liter. Levels higher than this cannot be sustained for prolonged periods of time.

Leadout   A tactic whereby a rider, usually a teammate, provides the benefit of a draft to better position another rider in the final moments before a sprint.

Lean Body Mass   Mass or weight without fat.

Leg Speed   How fast one can turn the cranks.

Mash   To push a big gear.

Mass-Start Races   Events in which riders start together from the same start line.

Motorpace   To draft a motorized vehicle. Often employed as a training technique. According to the vehicular code, illegal in many areas. Special safety precautions are advised.

Muffin Ride   Non-competitive supportive ride of friends with a muffin or pastry shop as a destination.

Noodle   To ride slowly.

Overtraining   Lack of fitness related to excessive intensity or duration of training. Mental or physical.

Oxygen Debt   Amount of oxygen used by the body during a recovery period from a work or interval period that is in excess of that used without work.

Paceline   Group of riders in a line, alternating turns pulling at the front and sitting in.

Peak   Good form, high physical fitness. Often the result of hard work combined with a period of good recovery.

Peloton   The main group of riders, the pack, field.

Periodization   Training different aspects of fitness at different periods of time.

Power   Work performed per unit of time.

Prime/Preme   An award given at selected points in a race. "A race within a race."

Pull   To ride into the wind without the benefit of a draft.

Pull Off   To move over and allow another to pull.

Pull Through   To assume the lead and take the wind.

Recovery   Period of training time when not working hard, rest period.

Repetitions   The number of times a task or interval is repeated.

Road Race In general, a race performed on paved surfaces. To be distinguished from a track or a mountain bike race.

Road races are divided specifically into criteriums, time trials, and road races. The specific road race is a mass-start event over a course more than one mile long. Road races may be point-to-point or circuits.

Rollers Stationary training device composed of three cyclindrical tubes (rollers) on which a bicycle sits.

Set In training, a group of repetitions.

Sew-up Integral tire and tube. The tube is sewn into the tire. Lighter and more responsive than a clincher tire. Also called a tubular.

Shelled Toasted. No pep left. Wasted.

Sit-in To rest, not pulling or working, to draft.

Snap The ability to accelerate quickly.

Specificity Training principle that states you specifically improve those characteristics of fitness that you work on while training.

Speed Quickness, how fast one can go.

Spin Often used to mean high cadence, it more accurately refers to the fluidity or suppleness of the pedal stroke.

Sprint Acceleration to speed.

Spun-out Unable to increase cadence, spinning as fast as possible. Implies the need for a bigger gear.

Squirrelly Riders who don't ride straight.

Stationary Trainer Training device that does not move. Rollers, Lifecycles, Turbo Trainers, and Trax stands are all varieties of stationary trainers.

Strategy Overall plan.

Strength Force that can be applied.

Tactic Action taken to further an overall strategy.

Tempo Pace. Normally implies hard, steady riding.

Toast Fried. Cooked. Well-done. Unable to ride any more.

Training Effort The body's response and adaptation to physical demands.

Turbo Trainer   Brand name of a type of stationary trainer device.

Volume of Training   Total time of intense training. If training is continuous, volume and duration are the same.

VO$_2$ Max   The maximum uptake of oxygen a person can utilize to produce energy. A measure of the ability of muscles to use oxygen. An important determinant of fitness and success.

Wind-up   To accelerate up to speed. Less abrupt than a jump, or attack.

For More Information

Bicycling Books

BICYCLING MEDICINE: HEALTH, FITNESS & INJURY EXPLAINED

Arnie Baker (San Diego, CA: Argo Publishing, 1995). Cycling health, fitness, and injury explained for riders and racers of all levels.

BICYCLE MAINTENANCE AND REPAIR

Bicycling Magazine (Emmaus, PA: Rodale Press, 1990).

THE BICYCLE WHEEL

Jobst Brandt (Menlo Park, CA: Avocet, 1981). Good information even if you don't build your own wheels.

CYCLING HEALTH AND PHYSIOLOGY

Edmund Burke (Brattleboro, VT: Vitesse Press, 1992). Physiology, nutrition, and training.

THE CYCLIST'S TRAINING BIBLE

Joe Friel (Boulder, CO: VeloPress, 1966). Comprehensive book on training for advanced racers.

HIGH-TECH CYCLING

Edmund Burke (Champaign, IL: Human Kinetics, 1996). Biomechanical, technical, and physiologic advances in cycling.

SCIENCE OF CYCLING

Edmund Burke (Champaign, IL: Human Kinetics, 1986). Good information on the scientific aspects of cycling.

SERIOUS CYCLING

Edmund Burke (Champaign, IL: Human Kinetics, 1995). Cycling training and performance.

BICYCLE ROAD RACING

Edward Borysewicz (Brattleboro, VT: Vitesse Press, 1985). Excellent though dated overview of road training and racing.

FITNESS CYCLING

Chris Carmichael and Edmund Burke (Champaign, IL: Human Kinetics, 1994). Basic training and programs for all levels.

EFFECTIVE CYCLING

John Forester (Cambridge, MA: The MIT Press, 1994). Bicycle advocacy: the bicyclist in traffic and society. Bicycle maintenance.

CYCLIST'S COMPANION

John Howard (Lexington, MA: Stephen Greene Press, 1984). Overview, somewhat dated.

COMPLETE BOOK OF BICYCLING

Greg LeMond (New York: G. P. Putnam's Sons, 1987). Basic training and tactics, interesting anecdotes.

ESSENTIAL TOURING CYCLIST

Richard Lovett (Camden, ME: Ragged Mountain Press, 1994). A complete course for the bicycle traveler.

BEGINNING BICYCLE RACING

Fred Matheny (Brattleboro, VT: Velo-news, 1987). Getting started, training methods, planning.

THE WOMAN CYCLIST

Elaine Mariolle and Michael Shermer (Chicago: Contemporary Books, 1988). Bicycling from a woman's perspective for women, with a section on this winning author's Race Across AMerica.

SOLO CYCLING

Fred Matheny (Brattleboro, VT: Velo-news, 1986). Good hints for time trialing, but dated.

WEIGHT TRAINING FOR CYCLISTS

Fred Matheny and Stephen Grabe (Brattleboro, VT: Velo-news, 1986). Photos and information about weight training for racers.

HEARTS OF LIONS

Peter Nye (New York: W. W. Norton, 1988). The story of American cycling heroes and racing.

TRAINING FOR CYCLING

David Phinney and Connie Carpenter (New York: Perigee, 1992). Training and tactics in racing.

FIT & FAST

Karen Roy and Thurlow Rogers (Brattleboro, VT: Vitesse, 1989). Training to be a better cyclist.

7/11 GRAND PRIX TRAINING MANUAL

Norma Sheil (Emmaus, PA: Rodale Press, 1982). Track training. Somewhat dated and hard to find.

SLOANE'S COMPLETE BOOK OF BICYCLING

Eugene Sloane (New York: Simon & Schuster, 1995). Overview, not limited to racing.

Books with Bicycling-Relevant Sections

STRETCHING

Bob Anderson (Bolinas, CA: Shelter Publications, 1980). A classic book on stretching.

THE ULTIMATE SPORTS NUTRITION HANDBOOK

Ellen Coleman (Palo Alto, CA: Bull Publishing, 1996). Solid, straightforward, accurate information.

THE HEART RATE MONITOR BOOK

Sally Edwards (Port Washington, NY: Polar CIC, 1992). Basics of heart-rate monitoring.

TRAINING LACTATE PULSE

Peter Janssen, G.J.M. (Oulu, Finland: Polar Electro Oy, 1987). Advanced concepts in heart-rate training.

GETTING STRONGER

Bill Pearl (Bolinas, CA: Shelter Publications, 1986). Weight lifting. Has a specific bicycling section.

SERIOUS TRAINING FOR SERIOUS ATHLETES

Rob Sleamaker (Champaign, IL: Leisure Press, 1989). Framework and philosophy of periodized training.

BEYOND TRAINING

Melvin H. Williams (Champaign, IL: Leisure Press, 1989). Legal and illegal enhancement.

Cycling Periodicals

BICYCLING

(33 E. Minor St., Emmaus, PA 18098). General interest.

BICYCLE GUIDE

(6420 Wilshire Blvd., Los Angeles, CA 90048). General interest.

BICYCLE USA

(190 W. Ostend St., Suite 120, Baltimore, MD 21230). League of American Wheelmen membership magazine.

CYCLING USA

(1 Olympic Plaza, Colorado Springs, CO 80909). United States Cycling Federation membership magazine.

MOUNTAIN BIKE ACTION

(25233 Anza Dr., Valencia, CA 91355). Mountain bike news; features on bikes and equipment.

PERFORMANCE CONDITIONING FOR CYCLING

(P. O. Box 6819, Lincoln, NB 68506). Newsletter dedicated to improving the cyclist.

VELONEWS

(1830 N. 55th, Boulder, CO 80301). Racing newspaper; training and equipment articles.

WINNING

(121 Second St., San Francisco, CA 94105). National and international racing.

Internet Newsgroups

PHL.BICYCLES

Bicycles, bike trails, recreation, and transportation.

REC.BICYCLES.MARKETPLACE

Buying, selling, and reviewing items for cycling.

REC.BICYCLES.MISC

General discussion of bicycling.

REC.BICYCLES.OFF-ROAD

All aspects of off-road bicycling.

REC.BICYCLES.RACING

Bicycle-racing techniques, rules, and results.

REC.BICYCLES.RIDES

Discussions of tours and training or commuting routes.

REC.BICYCLES.SOC

Societal issues of bicycling.

REC.BICYCLES.TECH

Cycling product design, construction, and maintenance.

Index

Lulling opponents into false sense of
security, 213–14

Macrocyles of training, 35
Magnetic resistance devices, 91
Maintenance of fitness level, 30
  aerobic, 55
Mass-start races, 155, 158
  see also specific types of races
Masters racing, 35, 158, 159
Mavic components, 16, 18
Maximum heart rate, 45–47
  in aerobic training, 54
  in stationary training, 108–9
  time trials and, 216
Mechanical accidents, 163
Medical causes of fatigue, 263–64
Medications, heart rate affected by, 50
Mental attitude, 233–44
  to avoid burnout, 236–37
  of champions, 238–39
  confident, 239–41
  optimistic, 244
  for time trials, 221–22
  visualization and, 242–44
  see also Motivation
Mesocyles of training, 35
Microcyles of training, 35
Millar, Robert, 238
Mishaps, 163
Mitochondria, 54, 56
Modifying workouts, 29
Montreal, University of, 228
Morning resting heart rate, 47
Moser, Francesco, 48
Motivation, 233–35
  heart-rate monitors and, 44
  stationary trainers and, 90
Mountain bike races, 156
Mouth, dry, 219
Multiple entries, 161
Mupirocin, 256
Muscle mass, maximum heart rate and,
  46
Muscles, post-race resting of,
  166

Myatt, Ralph, 92
Myosin, 56

National Off-Road Bicycle Association
  (NORBA), 155
National Public Radio (NPR), 238
Needs, hierarchy of, 234
Neosporin, 256
Nodules, subcutaneous, 257
Nolan, Margaret, 222
Noodling, 50
Nuke Proof components, 17
Numbers, racing, 162
  for time trials, 224
Nutrition, inadequate, 263
Nuts, lightweight, 19

Officials, racing, 164
Olympic Games, training for, 35–37
Optimal challenge or frustration, 234
Optimism, 244
Overconfidence, 240
Overtraining, 31
  fatigue due to, 263
Oxygen transport system, 55–56

Pacelines, 170
Pacing, 217, 226–28
Packs
  drafting in, 179
  dynamics of, 191
  echelons in, 170–71
  pacelines in, 170
  principles of riding in, 168–69
Passive blocking, 192
Pedals
  lightweight, 17
  rotation angle, 6–7
  safety check for, 10
Pedal-stroke emphasis, 34
Performance evaluation, 166
  after time trials, 221
Periodization, 30–31, 34–39
  annual chart, 38–39
  of weight training, 78–79
Perronnet, François, 228

Phinney, Davis, 197
Phosphocreatine, 41
Pilonidal sinus, blocked, 257
Placing, 164–65
Podium etiquette, 167
Points races, 156, 205
Polysporin, 256
Position, 5–8
  for attacks, 187
  crotchitis and, 261
  for time trials, 217, 218, 223
  training, 33
Power measurement, 33
Preparation for racing season, 37
Preregistration for races, 160
Primes, 204–7
Proactive riding, 181
Pro bike shops, 156
Pro Cycling, 155
Progress, measuring, 83–86
Progressive training, 29
Prophecies, self-fulfilling, 241
Proteins, 42–43
Protests of race results, 165
Proximity drills, 72
Psoriasis, 261
Pulling, 65
Pursuits, 156

Race Across America (RAAM), 155
Races, 153–84
  ability categories for, 159
  age and sex categories for, 158
  aggressive riding in, 181–82
  anticipation in, 180–81
  arriving at, 161–62
  bicycle clubs and, 157, 161
  bumping in, 172–73
  checking results of, 164–65
  cornering in, 176–79
  courses, 158
  energy conservation in, 182–84
  fees for, 161
  field limit for, 161
  group riding principles for, 168–69
  hand-ups in, 163–64

  hill technique for, 174–76
  mass-start, 158
  masters, 159
  mechanical accidents and mishaps
    during, 163
  mental factors in, see Mental attitude
  miles needed to train for, 157
  multiple entries in, 161
  numbers for, 162
  pacelines and echelons for, 169–71
  pro bike shops and, 156
  protests and appeals of results of,
    165
  registration for, 160
  role of officials in, 164
  rules for, 160
  sources of information on, 160
  things to do after, 165–67
  touching wheels in, 173
  types of, 155–56
  warming up for, 171–72
  women in, 159
  see also Criterium racing; Tactics,
    racing; Time trials
Range-of-motion adjustment, 20–22
Rash, road, 255–57
Records, training, 84–85
Recovery, 36–37
  annual pattern of, 38–39
  in interval training, 59
  measuring, 85–86
  after races, 165–66
Referees, 164
Regina components, 18
Registrars, 164
Registration for races, 160
Repeating workouts, 29
Repetitions in weight training, 76
Resistance devices, 91
Resting heart rate, 47–48
Results of races, checking, 164–66
Rims
  aerodynamic, 224
  gluing tubular or sew-up tires to, 12–
    15
  lightweight, 18

Touching wheels, 173
Tour de France, 197
Touring, 37
Track races, 156, 158
    primes in, 205
    registration for, 160
Track stand trainers, 90
Training, 29–43
    aerobic, 50–52, 54–56
    curve, 31–32
    energy systems and, 42–43
    excessive, 263
    fixed-gear, 68
    heart-rate monitoring during, 44–53
    leg strength and power work, 64–65
    leg-speed work, 62–64
    logs, 245–53
    measuring progress, 83–86
    miles needed for, 157
    periodized, 30–31, 34–39
    principles of, 29–31
    sprint, 65–67
    stretching, 72–74
    for time trials, 216
    with weaker rider, 68–72
    weekly schedule, 39–41
    workout variables, 32–34
    see also Anaerobic training; Interval training; Stationary trainers; Weight training
Trek bicycles, 15
Tricep curls, 82
TTT components, 17
Tubular tires, 12–15
    see also Sew-up Tires
Turnarounds, 218–19

Ulceration, 257
Ultimate components, 17, 19
Underconfidence, 240–41
United States Cycling Federation (USCF), 155, 159, 160

Upgrading, 159
USA Cycling, 155, 160

Vaginal infections, 262
Vaseline gauze, 256
Velodromes, 158
VeloMax components, 17
Visualization, 242–44
Vitus frameset, 16–17
VO_2 max, 228–29
Volume of training, 32

Warm–ups, 94
    before races, 171–72, 219–21
Water bottle cages
    lightweight, 18
    safety check for, 10
Water bottles for stationary training, 92
Weaker rider, training with, 68–72
Weight loss, excessive, 263
Weight of bicycle, reducing, 15–20
Weight training, 37, 66, 74–83
    annual pattern of, 39
    circuit, 77–78
    coaching philosophy in, 76
    determining how much to lift, 77
    exercises, 79–83
    logs, 250–53
    periodization of, 78–79
Wheels
    aerodynamic, 224
    safety check for, 8
    touching, 173
Wheelsuckers, 195–98
Winning (magazine), 238
Women, 158
    ability categories for, 159
    in clubs, 157
    crotchitis in, 259–62
    racing with men, 159
World Championships, 37, 197

Zipp components, 17